TRENDS AND ADVANCES IN LIVER DISEASES

Immunological, Metabolic and Infectious Aspects of Liver Transplantation

British Library Cataloguing in Publication Data
Immunological, metabolic and infectious aspects of liver transplantation.
 I. Vuitton, D.A.
 617.556

ISBN 086196-333-4

First published in 1991 by
John Libbey Eurotext
6, rue Blanche, 92120 Montrouge, France. (1) 47 35 85 52

John Libbey and Company Ltd
13, Smith Yard, Summerley Street, London SW18 4HR, England (1) 947 27 77

John Libbey CIC
Via Spallanzani 11, 00161, Rome, Italy

© John Libbey Eurotext, Paris, 1991. Il est interdit de reproduire intégralement ou partiellement le présent ouvrage – loi du 11 mars 1957 – sans autorisation de l'éditeur ou du Centre Français du Copyright, 6 bis rue Gabriel Laumain, 75010 Paris, France.

TRENDS AND ADVANCES IN LIVER DISEASES

Immunological, Metabolic and Infectious Aspects of Liver Transplantation

Proceedings of the International Congress
held in Chamrousse (France)
February, 1-2, 1991

This book has been published with the cooperation of Abbott, Duphar, Roche and Sandoz Laboratories

Editors

D.A. Vuitton
C. Balabaud
D. Houssin
D. Dhumeaux

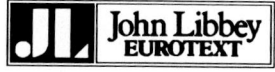

Contents

List of contributors VII
Foreword IX

The role of the major histocompatibility complex in the immune recognition and effector mechanism. *M.M. Tongio (Strasbourg, France)* 1

Study of graft rejection using molecular biology techniques. *C. Vanden Broecke, S. Caillat-Zucman, C. Legendre, L.H. Noël, H. Kreis, J.F. Bach, M. Tovey (Villejuif, Paris, France)* 11

Liver preservation - A review. *P. Bioulac-Sage, J. Carles, J.L. Gallis, G. Janvier, P. Canioni, C. Balabaud (Bordeaux, France)* 17

Liver transplantation - Immunological aspects of preservation and liver function. *G. Steinhoff (Hannover, Germany)* 27

The tolerance induced by liver allografting. *Y. Calmus, D. Houssin (Paris, France)* 35

Immunological indices of human liver allograft rejection. *D.H. Adams (Birmingham, UK)* 43

Cytological techniques in the follow-up of liver transplants. *K. Höckerstedt, I. Lautenschlager (Helsinki, Finland)* 49

Serum secretory component and plasma hyaluronic acid levels: complementary markers of graft rejection after liver transplantation ? *C. Vanlemmens, E. Seilles, D.A. Vuitton, B. Kantelip, S. Bresson-Hadni, J. Magnette, G. Mantion, M. Gillet, J.P. Miguet (Besançon, France)* 59

Prevention of hepatitis B virus (HBV) recurrence in liver transplant recipients by passive immunization. *R. Müller, G. Gubernatis, M. Farle, G. Niehoff, H. Klein, C. Wittekind, G. Tusch, H.U. Lautz, K. Böker, W. Stangel, R. Pichlmayr (Hannover, Germany)* 65

Contents

Incidence and prognosis of viral infections due to herpes viruses (other than cytomegalovirus), adenoviruses and hepatitis C virus in liver transplant recipients. *E. Dussaix (Le Kremlin-Bicêtre, France)* 77

Lymphoproliferative disorders in organ transplant recipients.
D. Cherqui (Créteil, France) 83

Recurrence of non-viral infectious diseases after liver transplantation.
S. Bresson-Hadni, D. Lenys, J.P. Miguet, D.A. Vuitton, M.C. Becker, G. Landecy, G. Mantion, M. Gillet (Besançon, France) 91

Does primary biliary cirrhosis recur after liver transplantation ? *J. Neuberger, S. Hubscher (Birmingham, UK)* 97

Author Index 107

List of contributors

Adams D.H., Selly Oak Hospital, Raddlebarn Road, Birmingham B29 6GD, United Kingdom.

Bioulac-Sage P. *et al.*, Service des Maladies de l'Appareil Digestif, Centre Hospitalier et Universitaire, Hôpital Saint-André, 1, rue Jean Burguet, 33075 Bordeaux, France.

Bresson-Hadni S. *et al.*, Service d'Hépatologie, Centre Hospitalier et Universitaire Jean Minjoz, Boulevard Fleming, 25030 Besançon Cedex, France.

Calmus Y. and Houssin D., Clinique Chirurgicale, Hôpital Cochin, 27, rue du Faubourg Saint-Jacques, 75674 Paris Cedex 14, France.

Cherqui D., Service de Chirurgie Générale et Digestive, Hôpital Henri Mondor, 51, avenue du Maréchal de-Lattre-de-Tassigny, 94010 Créteil Cedex, France.

Dussaix E., Laboratoire de Virologie, Centre Hospitalier et Universitaire de Bicêtre, 78, rue du Général Leclerc, 94275 Le Kremlin-Bicêtre Cedex, France.

Höckerstedt K. and Lautenschlager I., IV Department of Surgery, University of Helsinki, Surgical Hospital, Kasarmikatu 11-13, SF-00130 Helsinki, Finland.

Müller R. *et al.*, Abteilung für Gastroenterologie und Hepatologie, Medizinische Hochschule Hannover, Konstanty-Gutschow-Strasse 8, D-3000 Hannover 61, Germany.

Neuberger J. and Hubscher S., The liver and Hepatobiliary Unit, The Queen Elizabeth Hospital, Queen Elizabeth Medical Centre, Edgbaston, Birmingham B15 2TH, United Kingdom.

Steinhoff G., Klinik für Abdominal und Transplantations-chirurgie, Zentrum Chirurgie, Medizinische Hochschule Hannover, PO Box 610180, D-3000 Hannover 61, Germany.

Tongio M.M., Laboratoire d'Histocompatibilité, Centre Régional de Transfusion Sanguine de Strasbourg, 10, rue Spielmann, 67085 Strasbourg Cedex, France.

Vanden Broecke C. *et al.*, Centre d'Immunologie et de Biologie Parasitaire, Institut Pasteur, 1 rue du Professeur A. Calmette, BP 245, 59019 Lille, France.

Vanlemmens C. *et al.*, Service d'Hépatologie, Centre Hospitalier et Universitaire Jean Minjoz, Boulevard Fleming, 25030 Besançon Cedex, France.

Foreword

The French Association for the Study of the Liver has organized a special Seminar on "The immunological, metabolic and infectious aspects of liver transplantation" which was held February 1st and 2nd, 1991, at the ski resort in Chamrousse (France).
All the participants have found the program very enjoyable and the discussions very helpful. They asked us for the written text of the lectures, and suggested that a book be published. We thank John Libbey Eurotext Limited for having agreed to take on this project and the lecturers for having accepted to turn their lecture into a written form.
This seminar has taken place in a series of seminars which combine skiing and science and which are aimed at giving the "state of the art" on fundamental aspects of liver diseases. The first one was held in Chamrousse, in 1989, on "Cytoprotection and the liver". The next one will be held in 1992, on "Liver Regeneration".
We believe that the texts which are published in this book will be of help to the participants at the Seminar as well as to all those people who are interested in liver transplantation. We also hope that this book will become the first of a new series of books which will be able to give the "Trends and Advances in Liver Diseases" to every hepatologist who wants to get a comprehensive view of his speciality.

D.A. Vuitton
D. Dhumeaux

Immunological, metabolic and infectious aspects of liver transplantation. Eds D.A. Vuitton, C. Balabaud, D. Houssin, D. Dhumeaux. John Libbey Eurotext, Paris © 1991, pp. 1-10.

The role of the major histocompatibility complex in the immune recognition and effector mechanism

Marie-Marthe Tongio

Centre Régional de Transfusion Sanguine, 10 rue Spielmann, 67085 Strasbourg Cedex, France

To speak about the role of the Major Histocompatibility Complex in the immune recognition and effector mechanism, the three following points have to be considered. A. the recent knowledge about the human MHC system, B. the cells involved in the immune response where the MHC plays a role, C. the relationship existing between the HLA system and these cells.

A. THE HUMAN MHC SYSTEM

The major histocompatibility complex (MHC) in man, called HLA (Human Lymphocyte Antigen), was first discovered because of its role in the acceptance or rejection of transplants. It took several years to discover that its role was in fact more general and concerned the whole immune response.

1. The HLA system is polygenic. Several genes code for MHC molecules (Fig. 1).

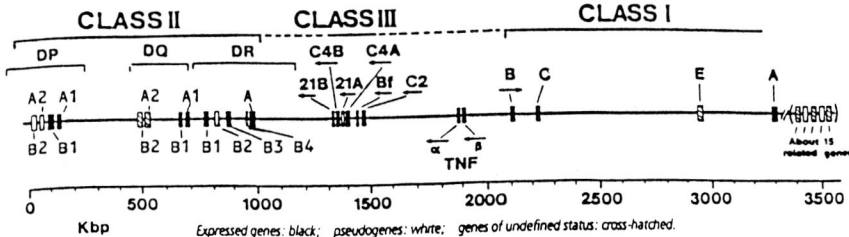

Fig 1 : Physical map of the human HLA region (according to J. Trowsdale and R.D. Campbell, Immunology Today 1988, 9 : 34).

a) class I genes (the classical HLA-A, B and C and the more recently found E, F and G genes) located telomeric on the short arm of chromosome 6 code for a 45 kilodalton (kd) α chain composed of three extracellular domains (α1, α2 and α3), a transmembrane part and an intracytoplasmic part. This class I α chain is non covalently associated with a 12 kd β 2 microglobulin chain which is necessary for class I antigenic expression (Fig. 2). Class I MHC molecules are expressed on nearly all nucleated cells.

b) class II genes are subdivided into DR, DQ and DP subregions (the DR subregion comprises a DRA and several DRB genes, the DQ subregion comprises DQ A1, B1, A2 and B2 genes and the DP subregion comprises DP A1, B1, A2 and B2 genes). Class II molecules are built of an ~ 34 kd α chain coded by a class IIA gene (DRA, DQA or DPA) and an ~ 28 kd β chain coded by a class II B gene (DRB1, B3, B4 or B5, DQ B and DP B). Both α and β chains are composed of two extracellular domains (respectively α1, α2 and β1, β2), a transmembrane part and an intracytoplasmic part. The α and β chains are non covalently associated (Fig. 2). Class II MHC molecules have a limited cellular distribution and are expressed on a few cell types, in particular dendritic cells, B lymphocytes, macrophages, endothelial cells and cutaneous Langerhans cells.

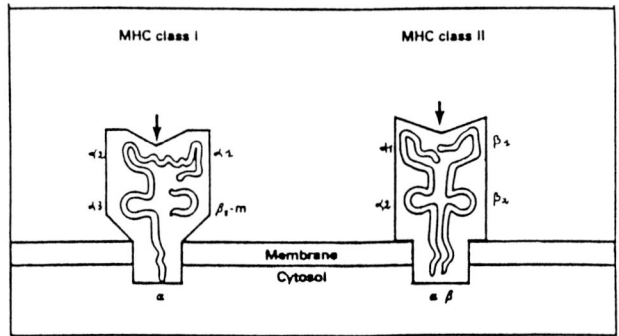

Fig. 2 : Structure of HLA class I and class II molecules (according to JM Austyn. Antigen presenting cells IRL Press, Oxford University Press, 1989).

2. The HLA system is polyallelic. Several alleles exist for the class I and class II DRB1, DQA1, DQB1, DPA1 and DPB1 genes, leading to the existence of 24 HLA-A, 50 HLA-B, 11 HLA-C, 18 HLA-DR, 9 HLA-DQ and 6 HLA-DP specificities (Table 1).

Table 1 :
Nomenclature for factors of the HLA system 1987 according to Human Immunology 1989, 26, 3-14.

A	B	C	DR	DQ	DP
A1	B5	Cw1	DR1	DQw1	DPw1
A2	B7	Cw2	DR2	DQw2	DPw2
A3	B8	Cw3	DR3	DQw3	DPw3
A9	B12	Cw4	DR4	DQw4	DPw4
A10	B13	Cw5	DR5	DQw5(w1)	DPw5
A11	B14	Cw6	DRw6	DQw6(w1)	DPw6
Aw19	B15	Cw7	DR7	DQw7(w3)	
A23(9)	B16	Cw8	DRw8	DQw8(w3)	
A24(9)	B17	Cw9(w3)	DR9	DQw9)(w3)	
A25(10)	B18	Cw10(w3)	DRw10		
A26(10)	B21	Cw11	DRw11(5)		
A28	Bw22		DRw12(5)		
A29(w19)	B27		DRw13(6)		
A30(w19)	B35		DRw14(6)		
A31(w19)	B37		DRw15(2)		
A32(w19)	B38(16)		DRw16(2)		
Aw34(10)	B39(16)		DRw17(3)		
Aw36	B40		DRw18(3)		
Aw43	Bw41				
Aw66(10)	Bw42		DRw52		
Aw68(28)	B44(12)				
Aw69(28)	B45(12)		DRw53		
Aw74(w19)	Bw46				
	Bw47				
	Bw48				
	B49(21)				
	Bw50(21)				
	B51(5)				
	Bw52(5)				
	Bw53				
	Bw54(w22)				
	Bw55(w22)				
	Bw56(w22)				
	Bw57(17)				
	Bw58(17)				
	Bw59				
	Bw60(40)				
	Bw61(40)				
	Bw62(15)				
	Bw63(15)				
	Bw64(14)				
	Bw65(14)				
	Bw67				
	Bw70				
	Bw71(w70)				
	Bw72(w70)				
	Bw73				
	Bw75(15)				
	Bw76(15)				
	Bw77(15)				

3. The tridimensional structure of the HLA molecules. The recent work of Bjorkman et al (1), who studied by cristallography the tridimensional structure of the HLA-A2 molecule, showed that class I MHC molecules form a groove 25 Å long by 10 Å wide by 11 Å deep between their α1 and α2 domains where they are able to present peptides (Fig. 3). A comparative study performed for MHC class II molecules by Brown et al (2) concluded that although the structure of class I and class II molecules is different (Fig. 2), class II molecules also show a groove between their α1 and β1 domains and hence present peptides like class I molecules. The specificity of the class I and class II molecules results from a few aminoacid substitutions at some places inside the α1 and α2 domains for class I molecules (Fig. 4), the β1 domain for DR and the α1 and β1 domains for DQ and DP (3).

Fig. 3   **Structure of HLA-A2**

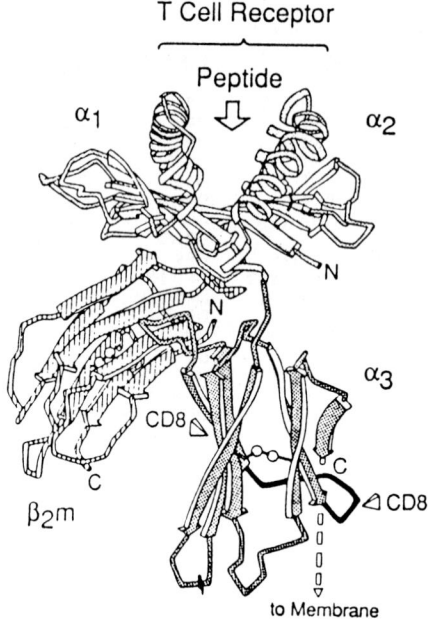

P. Parham, Scand J Rheumatology Suppl 87, p.13

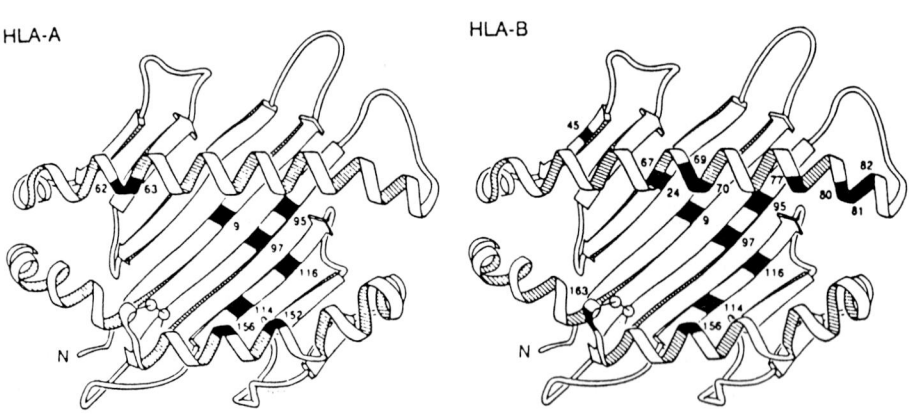

P. Parham, Scand J Rheumatology Suppl 87, p.17

Fig. 4 : Schematic diagram of the structure of the $\alpha 1$ and $\alpha 2$ domains showing the position of residues with variability greater or equal to 4 for HLA-A and HLA-B.

4. Peptides presented by the MHC molecules. Class I and class II MHC molecules do not present the same peptides. Class I molecules present "endogenous" peptides whereas class II molecules present "exogenous" peptides. Exogenous peptides result from the degradation of exogenous antigens (usually soluble foreign or self antigens), whereas endogenous peptides result from the degradation of antigens synthesized in the cell either by the cell DNA for self antigens or by a foreign viral DNA for example for foreign antigens. The pathways followed by the exogenous and endogenous antigens to be degraded into peptides are given in Fig. 5. Exogenous antigens are internalized by accessory cells like macrophages or cutaneous Langerhans cells. Once in the endosomes, they are degraded into small peptides (6-14 a.a) which associate with class II molecules. The class II molecules loaded with the exogenous peptides then migrate to the cell membrane. Endogenous antigens synthesized in the cell are degraded in the endoplasmic reticulum where they combine with class I molecules and migrate directly to the cell membrane. Endogenous peptides can usually not combine with class II molecules because class II molecules are associated, in the endoplasmic reticulum with a third class II chain called the invariant chain (different from the class II α and β chains) which hinders peptide association. More precise information about the endogenous peptide traffic (4) and the role of the invariant chain for class II presentation (5) has been published recently.

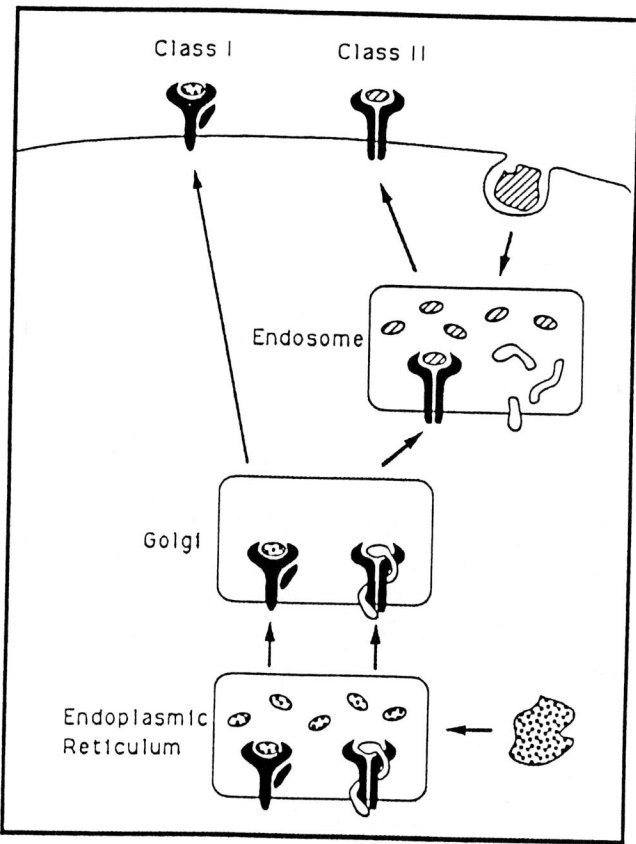

Fig. 5 Intracellular traffic and antigen processing. Different shadings have been used to represent MHC class I and class II molecules (black), invariant chain (white), exogenous antigen and fragments thereof (hatched), and endogenous antigen and fragments thereof (dotted). All elements are drawn schematically without any implication on their exact molecular structures

From E.O. Long, Immunology Today 1989, 10:232

B. CELLS INVOLVED IN THE IMMUNE RESPONSE

Three types of cells are involved in the immune response where HLA plays a role : accessory cells like dendritic cells, Langerhans cells and macrophages, B lymphocytes and T lymphocytes.

1. Accessory cells : macrophages and Langerhans cells can phagocyte and degrade particles via membrane receptors like Fc and complement receptors. Dendritic cells are composed of several different cell types whose localization differs (Table 2).

Table 2 Distribution of dendritic leukocytes

Type	Localization
Lymphoid dendritic cell (DC)	(Cells isolated from lymphoid tissues and studied *in vitro*)
Interdigitating cell (IDC)	T cell areas of secondary lymphoid tissues, and thymus medulla
Follicular dendritic cell (FDC)	B cell areas of secondary lymphoid tissues
Veiled cells (VC)	Afferent lymphatics, MNLX TDL (see text)
Langerhans cells (LC)	Epidermis of skin
Non-lymphoid or interstitial dendritic leukocytes	Interstitial connective tissue of most non-lymphoid organs

In : Austin, IRL Press 1989

2. B lymphocytes carry IgM immunoglobulins anchored in their membrane. Once a B cell has encountered the antigen for which it carries the specific anchored immunoglobulin, it becomes activated, follows clonal expansion and finally develops into a plasma cell which secretes soluble antibodies.

3. T lymphocytes are subdivided functionally into helper (Th) (usually CD4+), cytotoxic (Tc) and suppressor (Ts) (usually CD8+) subsets. T lymphocytes carry T cell receptors (TCRs) which can be one of two types ($\alpha\beta$ heterodimers which are the most frequent or $\gamma\delta$ heterodimers present on less than 10% of T lymphocytes). This paper will only refer to T lymphocytes carrying $\alpha\beta$ TCRs. These lymphocytes which migrate into the periphery have been previously selected in the thymus and represent only 5% of the total number of lymphocytes originally present in the thymus. They carry $\alpha\beta$ TCRs which recognize foreign antigens when they are presented by the self MHC molecules (a phenomenon called T cell restriction), but do not recognize self molecules presented by the MHC molecules.

T lymphocytes (Th or Tc) are subdivided into two categories - naive T lymphocytes which have never encounted an antigen and memory T lymphocytes which have already been sensitized. As will be seen later memory T lymphocytes can be activated by unique contact with the peptide presented by the self MHC, whereas naive T lymphocytes need in addition to contact with the peptide presented by the self MHC a second signal which can be the help provided by a cytokine or an adhesion molecule. This second signal depends highly on the accessory cell which presents the peptide with its self MHC.

C. RELATIONSHIP EXISTING BETWEEN THE HLA SYSTEM AND CELLS INVOLVED IN THE IMMUNE RESPONSE

The major function of the HLA system is to present self and foreign structures on or to cells involved in the immune response. The immune cooperation between the three cell types described above can be schematically summarized as follows (Fig. 6).

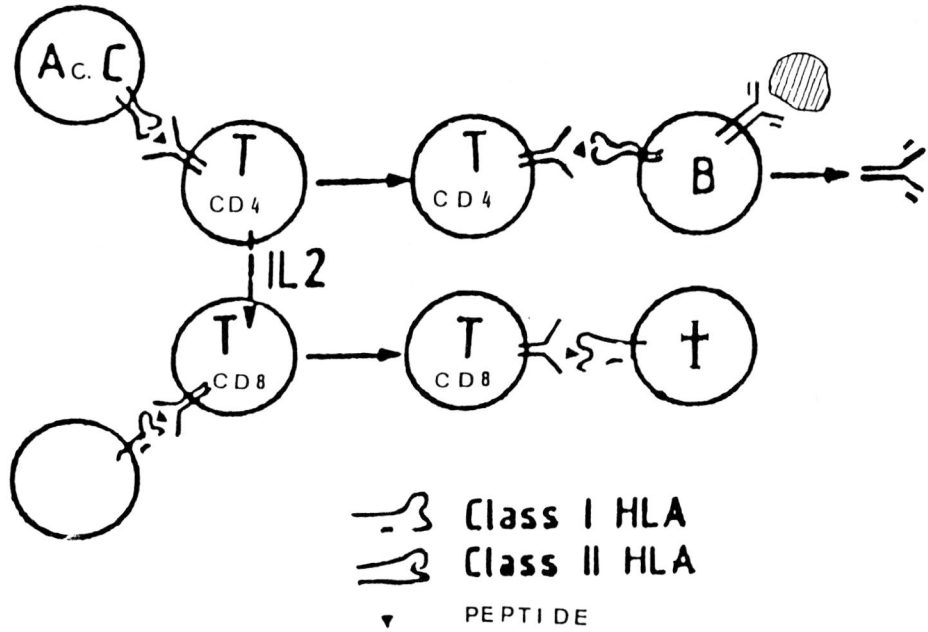

Fig. 6

Accessory cells internalize exogenous antigens (self or foreign) and present the degraded peptides with their class II molecules (6). Depending on the specificity carried by the MHC class II molecules, some peptides will be selected and presented and others not.

- Not only macrophages, but also B cells, are capable of internalizing foreign antigens. This internalization is very specific since only B lymphocytes carrying an anchored immunoglobulin specific for the native antigen will internalize the antigen using the immunoglobulin as an antigen receptor. Antigen degradation into peptides will occur and selected peptides will be re-expressed on the membrane of the B cells in association with class II molecules.

- T α β receptors of Th cells recognize the foreign peptide-class II complex on accessory cells and on B lymphocytes when the T lymphocytes are memory cells. This recognition results in secretion by the Th cells of antigen non specific mediators which activate :

1) macrophages, by secretion by the Th cells of Interferon γ (IFNγ).
2) B lymphocytes, by secretion by the Th cells of Interleukin 2 (IL2) and Interleukin 6 (IL6). Once activated, B lymphocytes develop into plasma cells and secrete soluble antibodies which recognize the native protein.
3) Tc lymphocytes, by secretion by the Th cells of IL-2 and Interleukin 4 (IL-4). Once activated, the resting Tcs become effector Tcs. The α β TCRs of these effector Tc lymphocytes then recognize processed foreign peptides bound to MHC class I molecules.

As a schematic summary, Th lymphocytes recognize foreign peptides presented by self class II molecules. These peptides result from the degradation of exogenous molecules in endosomes. Tc lymphocytes recognize foreign peptides presented by self class I molecules. These peptides result from the degradation of endogenous molecules in the endoplasmic reticulum (7). Class I molecules being expressed on nearly all nucleated cells, all these cells are susceptible to become targets for Tc cells when expressing a viral foreign antigen with their class I molecules for example.

When the T lymphocytes are naive T cells recognition of the MHC molecule loaded with a peptide is not sufficient to activate them. A second signal is required. Dendritic accessory cells are capable of bringing this second signal and are thus particularly potent activators of naive cells. When naive T cells encounter other accessory cells which are not able to bring a second signal, the T cells instead of becoming activated will become tolerant. Thus depending on the accessory cells which present the peptide, naive T cells will become either activated or tolerant (Fig. 7).

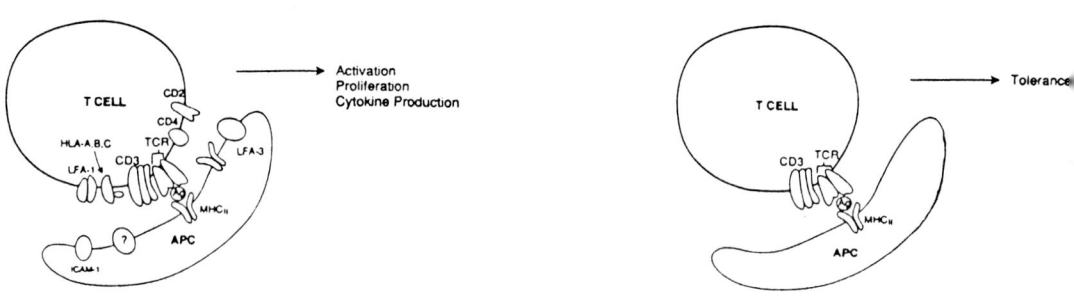

Model of tolerance induction induced by antigen recognition in the absence of appropriate AC co-stimulation

Geppert et al., Immunological Reviews 1990, 117:5

Fig. 7

All these data refer to the immune response restricted by the self MHC molecules. How then can one explain alloreactivity ? Two mechanisms have to be considered (Fig. 8).

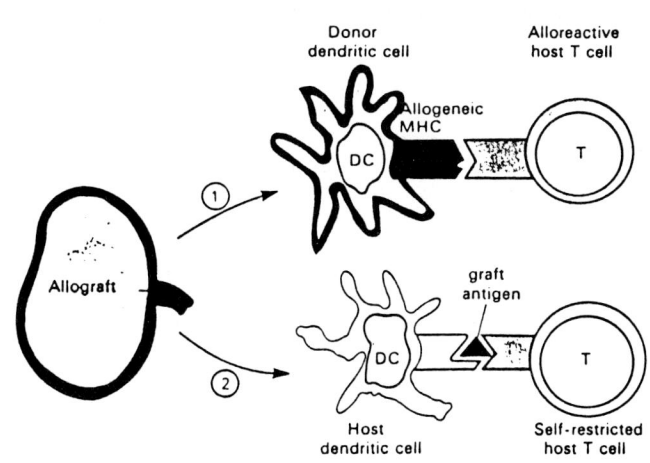

Figure 8   Routes for sensitization of recipients to graft antigens. (**Route 1**) Dendritic cells from the graft present their own MHC molecules to alloreactive T cells. (**Route 2**) Host dendritic cells present processed graft antigens to self-restricted T cells.
In : Austin, IRL Press 1989

The first one is classical and fits MHC restriction. Foreign antigens provided by the graft are processed by the host cells and presented by dendritic cells. Autologous T cells can thus be activated. The second mechanism remains in part unexplained. Foreign dendritic cells present their MHC antigens or peptides presented by their MHC antigens to the T cell receptors of the host. T cell stimulation results although the TCRs of the T cells have been educated to recognize "only foreign peptides presented by the self MHC". Several hypotheses have been put forward to try to explain this phenomenon without conclusive results.

REFERENCES

1. Bjorkmann, P.J., Saper, M.A., Samraoui, B., Bennet, W.S., Strominger, J.L., Wiley, D.C. (1987) : Structure of the human class I histocompatibility antigen, HLA-A2. Nature 329: 506-512.

2. Brown, J.H., Jardetzky, T., Saper, M.A., Samraoui, B., Bjorkmann, P.J., Wiley, D.C. (1988) : A hypothetical model of the foreign antigen binding site of class II histocompatibility molecules. Nature 332: 845-850.

3. Marsh, S.G.E., Bodmer, J.D. (1989) : HLA-DR and -DQ epitopes and monoclonal antibody specificity. Immunology Today 10 : 305.

4. Parham, P. (1990) : Transporters of delight. Nature 348 : 674.

5. Brodsky, F.M. (1990) : The invariant dating service. Nature 348 : 581.

6. Unanue, E.R., Allen, P.M. (1987) : The basis for the immunoregulatory role of macrophages and other accessory cells. Science 236 : 551-557.

7. Lippincott-Schwartz, J., Bonifacino, J.S., Yuan, L.C., Klausner, R.F. (1988) : Degradation from the endoplasmic reticulum : disposing of newly synthesized proteins. Cell 54 : 209-220.

Study of graft rejection using molecular biology techniques

Catherine Vanden Broecke[1][3], Sophie Caillat-Zucman[2], Christophe Legendre[2], Laure-Hélène Noël[2], Henri Kreis[2], Jean-François Bach[2], Michael Tovey[1]

[1] *Laboratoire d'Oncologie virale, IRSC-CNRS, Villejuif, France.* [2] *INSERM U25 et Département de Néphrologie, Hôpital Necker, Paris, France,* [3] *Present address : Centre d'Immunologie et de Biologie Parasitaire. INSERM U167-CNRS 624, Institut Pasteur, Lille, France*

Abstract

Several cytokines which play an important role as mediators in the regulation of the immune system are thought to be involved in processes such as allograft rejection. Cytokines generally function at low concentrations and locally at the site of rejection. Thus, the assays of cytokines in blood or urine only give very imprecise indication of their levels at the site of rejection and, consequently, provide only limited informations for comprehension of the mechanisms involved in rejection. Therefore, highly sensitive methods were developed using the techniques of molecular biology to detect the expression of cytokine genes at the site of graft rejection. Northern blot analysis was used to study the messenger RNA (mRNA) coding for different cytokines in several experimental models of cardiac and renal graft rejection. Such methods require too much tissular material it to be applied in human studies. The Polymerase Chain Reaction (PCR), however, allows the detection of as low as one copy of mRNA in samples of human tissues. These two techniques do not give, however, any information on the cellular origin of cytokine gene expression.

In order to study human renal graft rejection, we developed a highly sensitive method of *in situ* hybridization based on the use of 35S labelled riboprobes. We have studied at the cellular level the production of the mRNA of different cytokines in renal biopsies from normal individuals, patients undergoing a first episode of kidney allograft rejection or patients without evidence of kidney allograft rejection. Our main observation is that the gene for Il-6 but not IFNγ is expressed at time of rejection by all cellular types. The chronological analysis of cytokine gene expression (including other cytokines like TNF, IL-2 ...) is underway.

INTRODUCTION

Recent studies have shown that allograft rejection is a complex process involving the action of specific effector T cells, non specific effector cells (natural killer (NK), lymphokine activated killer (LAK)) and non specific soluble factors (Mason et al.; 1984). In particular, soluble factors play a key role in cooperation between allosensitized cells and effector cells leading to allograft rejection. Cytokines such as TNF-α, IL-1 and IL-6 have been shown to be produced during graft rejection as determined by Elisa tests or the measurement of biological activities in different body fluids (blood, urine...) (Maury & Peppo, 1987; Van Oers et al., 1988; Maury & Teppo, 1987). The analysis of the presence of cytokines in biological fluids provides only indirect evidence, however, for changes in a particular organ. Indeed cytokines function primarily over limited distances and at very low concentrations. The absence of detection of cytokines in fluids could also be due to the low sensitivity of some biological assays and would therefore give an incorrect idea of changes in the level of cytokines at the site of graft rejection. Moreover, an increase of cytokine production in body fluids due to rejection can only with difficulty be distinguished from other causes such as infection or graft dysfunction. Therefore technical means available to evaluate minimal local modifications of cytokine production during graft rejection needed established.

The development of the techniques of molecular biology has allowed the study of modifications of the expression of cytokine genes by the determination of changes of mRNA levels in tissue and organs.

MOLECULAR BIOLOGY TECHNIQUES IN GRAFT REJECTION : ADVANTAGES AND DISADVANTAGES

Three principle techniques have been applied to the study of changes in cytokine gene expression during graft rejection : Northern Blot analysis, polymerase chain reaction (PCR) and *in situ* hybridization.Their main characteristics, advantages and disadvantages are now described in Table 1.

Northern blot analysis

The Northern blot technique consists in separating mRNAs present in an organ extract on a denaturing agarose gel, which are then transferred on a nylon or nitrocellulose membrane. Specific transcripts for a particular cytokine are revealed by hybridization of the membrane with the appropriate radio- or chemically labelled probes (DNA or RNA). Until now, it has been successfully applied in experimental animal models (mouse and rat cardiac allografts and rat renal allograft) (Lowry & Blais, 1988; Dallman et al., 1989; Lowry et al., 1989). An early and transient expression of IL-2, TNF-α and IFN-γ has been observed in allogeneic grafts approximately five days after mouse cardiac transplantation. No difference was observed in the expression of these cytokines when animals were rendered tolerant prior to grafting or when animals received a syngeneic graft.

Northern blot analysis has two major disadvantages. Firstly, the technique requires relatively large quantities of total or poly A+ RNA and consequently relatively large amounts of tissue and can only with difficulty be applied to studies in man. Secondly, Northern blot analysis does not provide information on the cellular localization of cytokine gene expression.

Table 1 : Major advantages and disadvantages of molecular biology techniques used for the study of graft rejection

	Sensitivity of the method	Localization of cytokine gene expression	Applicable to human biopsies
Northern blot	++	no	no
Polymerase Chain Reaction (PCR)	+++	no	yes
In situ Hybridization	+++	yes	yes

Polymerase Chain Reaction (PCR)

The Polymerase Chain Reaction (PCR) has been used in the study of graft rejection in experimental models, mainly by Dallman et al., 1991. Briefly, the method is based on the principle of amplification of cDNA synthesized with a reverse transcriptase from cytokine mRNA present in the sample studied using two appropriate oligonucleotide primers. The PCR products are separated on an agarose gel, blotted on a nylon membrane and hybridized with a specific internal labelled oligonucleotide. This technique, which only needs minimal material, is more sensitive than the Northern blot analysis as it is capable of detecting as little as one copy of mRNA. The work of Dallman revealed that cytokine genes are transcribed differentially during mouse graft rejection. Some cytokine genes are expressed only following the grafting of tissue while other cytokines are expressed in both syngeneic and allogeneic tissue or even in non grafted tissue.

Local analysis of cytokine production during human graft rejection requires the application of the technique on biopsies from transplantation patients. Although conventionnal PCR analysis can be used to study cytokine expression in human biopsies, the technique does not allow however the cellular localization of gene expression. On the contrary, we have developed in our laboratory a highly sensitive technique of in situ hybridization able to localize on biopsy sections the expression of different cytokine genes in individual cells (Vanden Broecke et al., 1991a,b).

In situ Hybridization

In comparison to the two techniques described previously, the main advantage of the *in situ* hybridization is the conservation of tissue histology which allows direct cellular localization and characterization of specific gene expression (Lum, 1986). By using an antisens (35)S labelled RNA probe of vey high specific activity, we have developed a technique of *in situ* hybridization capable of detecting as few as 1 to 5 copies of a cytokine messenger RNA in individual cells. This technique allowed us to study the expression of several cytokines (IL-6, IFNγ and TNF-α) during human renal graft rejection. Three groups of patients were included in the experiment :

group 1= 5 patients without histologic evidence of kidney disease
group 2= 5 kidney transplant patients without evidence of rejection
group 3= 8 kidney transplant patients undergoing a first episode of acute rejection in the first two months following transplantation.

The technique and the results which have been described in detail elsewhere (Vanden Broecke et al., 1991b), are briefly reported here. μm sections from 4% paraformaldehyde fixed-paraffin embedded kidney biopsies from the 18 subjects were hybridized for 16 hours at 50°C in the presence of 40 pg/μl of a cytokine specific antisense (35S) RNA probe in 50% formamide. Following hybridization, sections were treated with RNase A to remove the unhybridized probe, washed in stringent conditions to eliminate non specific hybridization, coated in photographic emulsion, developed after ±10 days and stained appropriately. Labelling was considered to be specific when the mean number of silver grains obtained on the section with the labelled probe was reduced by at least 2.5 fold when similar hybridization was performed in the presence of a 200 fold excess of the specific unlabelled probe.

No IL-6, IFNγ or TNF-α transcript was revealed in the biopsies from human normal kidney or from kidneys from transplanted patients with stable renal function (except one case). On the contrary, significant levels of Il-6 mRNA but not IFNγ or TNF-α were present in all cellular types of renal biopsies from 6 of 8 kidney transplanted patients with a first episode of rejection (group 3). In one patient of group 3, for which no IL-6 had been detected, juxtatubular clusters of grains revealing the presence of TNF-α were observed. As it is known that TNF-α, among other cytokines, is a potent inducer of IL-6, this results can be interpretated as due to different kinetics of production of these cytokines. In the same way, the absence of detection of IFNγ transcripts in samples of tissues of transplantation patients undergoing a kidney rejection could be explained by an earlier and transient expression of this cytokine.

PERSPECTIVES

Undoubtly, The *in situ* hybridization technique brings essential informations on cytokine production during acute allograft rejection such as local detection of the presence of low levels of cytokine transcripts (also given by PCR) and cellular localization of the gene expression. More precise information about cytokine production during acute rejection will be provided in the future by the combination of *in situ* hybridization and immunocytochemistry, thus allowing the immunological characterization of cytokine gene expressing cells. *In situ* hybridization has also the advantage, shared by PCR but not by Northern Blotting, of being applicable in the study of human allograft rejection by the analysis of biopsy sections. The analysis by *in situ* hybridization and PCR of serial biopsies taken regularly from the day of transplantation will therefore bring direct information on the local cascade of cytokine production prior and at the time of rejection, which will contribute to our understanding of the processes which lead to human allograft rejection.

REFERENCES

Dallman,M.J. et al. (1989): Lymphokine production in allografts. Analysis of RNA by Northern Blotting. *Transplantation Proceedings* 21, 296-298.

Dallman,M.J. et al. (1991): Cytokine gene expression : analysis using Northern Blotting, Polymerase Chain Reaction and *in situ* Hybridization. *Immunol. Rev.* 119, 163-179.

Lowry,R.P. and Blais, D. (1988): Tumor necrosis factor-alpha in rejecting rat cardiac allografts. *Transplantation Proceedings* 20, 245-247.

Lowry,R.P. et al. (1989) Lymphokine transcription in vascularized mouse heart grafts : effect of "tolerance" induction. *Transplantation proceedings* 21, 72-73.

Lum,J.B. (1986) Visualization of mRNA transcription of specific genes in human cells and tissues using *in situ* hybridization. *Bio Techniques* 4, 32-39.

Mason,D.W. et al. (1984): Mechanisms of allograft rejection. The role of cytotoxic T-cells and delayed-type-hypersensitivity. *Immunol. Rev.* 77, 167-184

Maury,C.P.J. and Teppo,A.-M. (1987): Raised serum levels of cachetin/tumor necrosis factor α in renal allograft rejection. *J. Exp. Med.* 166; 132-137.

Maury,C.P.J. and Teppo,A.-M. (1988): Serum immunoreactive interleukin 1 in renal transplant recipients. *Transplantation* 45, 143-146.

Vanden Broecke,C.and Tovey, M.G.(1991a) Expression of the genes of class I interferons and Interleukin-6 in individual cells. *J. IFN Research* 11, 91-103.

Vanden Broecke,C. et al. (1991b): Differential in situ expression of cytokines in renal allograft rejection. *Transplantation* 51, 602-609.

Van Oers,M.H.J. et al.(1988): Interleukin 6 (IL-6) in serum and urine of renal transplant recipients. *Clin. Exp. Immunol.* 71, 314-319.

Immunological, metabolic and infectious aspects of liver transplantation. Eds D.A. Vuitton, C. Balabaud, D. Houssin, D. Dhumeaux. John Libbey Eurotext, Paris © 1991, pp. 17-26.

Liver preservation - A review

Paulette Bioulac-Sage*, Jacques Carles, Jean-Louis Gallis, Gérard Janvier, Paul Canioni, Charles Balabaud

Laboratoire des Interactions Cellulaires et laboratoire de RMN-IBCN, CNRS, Université de Bordeaux II, 146 rue Léo-Saignat, 33076, Bordeaux. Centre de transplantation, CHU Pellegrin, 33076 Bordeaux, France

* Author for correspondence

INTRODUCTION

The introduction of Belzer University of Wisconsin (UW) cold storage solution into clinical transplantation (T) has revolutionized nearly all aspects of liver T today (table 1) (Belzer et al 1988). Many of the reasons why this solution is effective have recently been reviewed (Southard et al 1990). In studies on the rat it has been shown that after 24 h or 48 h storage in Euro-Collins (EC) solution, although virtually all parenchymal cells remained viable, severe damage was observed to non-parenchymal cells (NPC) and about 40% of NPC were trypan blue positive (Caldwell-Kenkel 1989). It is therefore important to pay special attention to the anatomy and function of these cells (fig. 1 and table 2) and to understand the interplay between blood, NPC and hepatocytes.
There are several methods for studying the efficiency of preservation, the ultimate being orthotopic liver transplantation (OLT) (table 3). It must also be kept in mind that preservation in clinical practice is a multifactorial process beginning in the donor and finishing in the recipient and cannot be dissociated

Table 1. Percentage survival (%), beyond 5-7 days, after orthotopic liver transplantation performed in different species according to the length of preservation in UW

HOURS	RAT	DOG	HUMAN
0 h	94[1,2]		
9 h	56	10 (EC)	
12 h		100	100
24 h	100[3] 63[2]		100?
30 h	50[3]		
48 h		83	
72 h		87[4]	

[1]Sprague Dawley,[2]Wistar,[3]Wag,[4]Machine perfusion(gluconate)(Pienaar et al 1990), EC:Euro-Collins

from medical history of each (table 4).In this short and very schematic review we shall focus on 4 main areas:

1- NMR studies of intracellular pH and energetic metabolism.

2- Reperfusion injury.

3- The morphology of sinusoidal cells

4- The interplay between liver donor, preservation injury and rejection.

Table 2. Main functions of sinusoidal endothelial and Kupffer cells

ENDOTHELIAL CELLS
* The main structural element of the wall of liver sinusoids.
* Functions :
   - FILTRATION (numerous fenestrations +++ = 100 nm diameter)
   - ENDOCYTOSIS (numerous micropinocytic vesicles - endosomes - lysosomes) : major components of connective tissue, lysosomal enzymes... are eliminated rapidely and almost exclusively from the blood by receptor - mediated endocytosis in the EC.
   - SYNTHESIS OF EFFECTOR MOLECULES (capable of modifying the function of other cells): various eicosanoids (PGE_2 , prostacyclin $\longrightarrow$ vasodilatation...), angiotensin - converting enzyme, other signal molecules ...
   - ENERGY METABOLISM
        numerous enzyme activities:lysosomal, energy metabolism enzymes ...
   - Play an active role in the IMMUNOBIOLOGICAL system of the liver (endothelial adhesion molecules)

KUPPFER CELLS (KC)
* Main cells of the Mononuclear Phagocytic System (80-90 % of fixed macrophages)
* Presenting Ag-cell (participate in the immunobiological system of the liver)
* Functions :
   - ENDOCYTOSIS (numerous and various types of lysosomes)
      Pinocytosis, Phagocytosis
   - NUMEROUS SECRETORY PRODUCTS:
mediators: IL-1, 6, TNF α β, IFN α, PDGF, FGF, TGF α β, IGF 1..., complement components, coagulation factors, proteolytic enzymes, enzyme inhibitors, colony-stimulating factors..., ECM or cell adhesion proteins (fibronectin,heparan sulfate proteoglycan...)
   - KC are involved in the clearance of immune complexes, the inflammatory process, immune response...
* Numerous factors or signals modulate the functions of Kupffer Cells

   ACTIVATED KC cause a chain reaction (release of mediators, lysosomal enzymes, production of superoxide...)
* There are 3 types of Kupffer Cells
   - Macrophages with no contact with a stimulator
   - Primed macrophages : exposed to immunological stimulation
   - Activated macrophages:primed macrophages, subsequently exposed to a trigger
     signal (ex: endotoxin...)

Fig.1.Schematic representation of a liver sinusoid and sinusoidal cells.

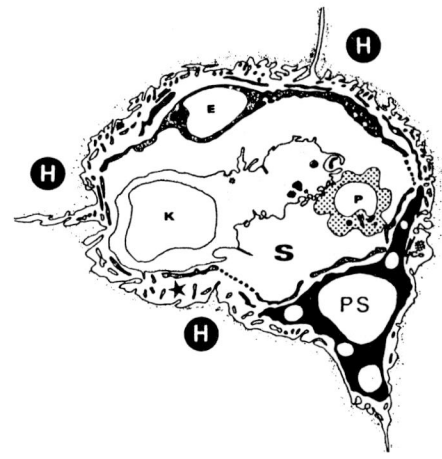

Sinusoidal volume : 21.8% of hepatic parenchyma, sinusoidal lumen (S): 10.6%, Disse space (star): 4.9 %, Sinusoidal cells (SC): 6.3% (26.5 % of plasma membrane surface).
Endothelial cells (E): 44 % of SC.Kupffer cells (K): 32 % of SC. Perisinusoidal cells (PS):13 % of SC.The Disse space contains the extracellular matrix: a- Proteins with collagens (I,III,IV,VI) and elastin, b- Glycoconjugates with structural glycoproteins (fibronectin, laminin, undulin, nidogen, tenascin) and proteoglycans (heparan sulfate, dermatan sulfate, chondroitine 4-sulfate), c- Glycosaminoglycan (hyaluronate)
H: Hepatocyte; P:Pit cell

Table 3. Methods for the study of liver preservation

ORTHOTOPIC LIVER TRANSPLANTATION (survival)- MICROCIRCULATION (microcinema)- NMR- ISOLATED RAT LIVER PERFUSION :
- Bile production - Vascular resistance - Microcirculation
- Liver enzymes: Hepatocytes (ASAT, ALAT). Endothelial (purine nucleoside phosphorylase, CPK). Kupffer (cytokines, proteases etc...)
- Cell viability (trypan blue) - Histology : light microscopy, electron microscopy, immunohistochemistry
- Metabolic functions:energy,oxydative metabolism (generation of free radicals)

Table 4. Factors involved in human graft viability

POTENTIAL DONOR	OLT	RECIPIENT
Nutritional status	Harvesting (Procurement)	Immunology[1]
Liver disease	Cold preservation (ischemia)	Endotoxinemia
Hemodynamic instability	Reperfusion injury	Liver disease[2]
	Technical problems[3]	Hemodynamic instability

[1] (ABO, preformed lymphocytotoxic Ab, positive cross match)   [2] (BS, bil, toxins)   [3] (Artery[+++], PV, VC, Bile duct[++])
PV: portal vein, VC: vena cava, BS: bile salts, Bil: bilirubin

I - NMR STUDIES OF INTRACELLULAR pH AND ENERGETIC METABOLISM.

P-31 NMR is an ideal method for the non-invasive and non-destructive observation and monitoring of energetic metabolites in tissues. From analysis of the recorded spectra, it is possible to quantify the content of "NMR visible" ATP, ADP and inorganic phosphate (Pi) in the perfused liver. In addition, the chemical shift of Pi is pH dependent and the position of the Pi resonance in the spectrum leads to the determination of cytosolic pH (Desmoulin et al., 1987). Two preservation solutions have proved their efficiency in human liver transplantation :EC, with low sodium (10 mM), high potassium (115 mM) plus high glucose content (200 mM) , and UW with low sodium (30 mM), high potassium (125 mM) and high lactobionate (100 mM) content.Recently, Bretschneider's solution (HTK solution) has been found to effectively preserve the kidney and the liver of experimental animals (Holzmueller et al., 1990). The characteristic of this solution is its low sodium

and potassium content (15-10 mM), and high histidine concentration (200mM).
We used the P-31 NMR technique for monitoring changes in the metabolic state and intracellular pH of the excised perfused rat liver subjected to phases of hypothermic perfusion and prolonged cold ischemia, followed by normothermic reperfusion. Nucleoside triphosphate (NTP) depletion and intracellular pH (pHin) were studied over an 18-24 h cold (4°C) storage period, using three preservation media: EC, UW and HTK. Values obtained after 8 h ischemia were selected to estimate the performance of the various media and ischemic damage was assessed by reperfusing the stored organ with Krebs medium. pHin reached values of 7.15±0.10 in UW and HTK, and 6.96±0.10 in EC-stored livers. Recovery of pHin was near the control value (7.23±0.08), except for EC solution (7.05±0.20). Even though hepatic NTP levels were much higher in UW-treated livers (37±7%) than in other groups (HTK:10±5% and EC:0% of control levels), NTP recovery was unexpectly similar (around 70±20%) between the groups on reperfusion. Post-ischemic NTP recovery is generally considered a good index of liver viability. Yet the maximum storage period followed by animal survival after transplantation was 12 h with EC (Howden et al., 1990). Results should be analysed taking into account thermic changes during post-ischemic reperfusion. In a complementary study (Fig.2), 24 h HTK or UW-preserved rat liver was reperfused using Krebs-Henseleit medium, at 4°C for the first 20 min and then at 37°C (for at least 30 min). At the onset of the hypothermic reflush, there was an immediate recovery of hepatic ATP levels, reaching similar levels for both solutions: 77±11% (UW) and 66±5% (HTK) within 20 min, and, likewise for both, a rapid increase of pHin. Changing the temperature from 4°C to 37°C induced a further recovery of ATP levels (HTK:95±11% and UW:90±5%). Throughout the subsequent warm perfusion, even though pHin was maintained at physiological values (7.21±0.09), for both solutions, NTP levels in UW-preserved livers remained constant whereas they decreased in HTK-preserved livers. Since there is no allopurinol in HTK, the latter effect might in part be due to the deleterious action of free radicals generated as a result of thermic stress. On the other hand, reflushed HTK-stored liver showed a residual high content of intracellular histidine (as we have observed with proton-decoupled C-13 NMR) which can lead to glutamate and glutamine production. This, in turn, can activate glycogen synthesis which causes an increase in the consumption of the energetic metabolites such as UTP and ATP.

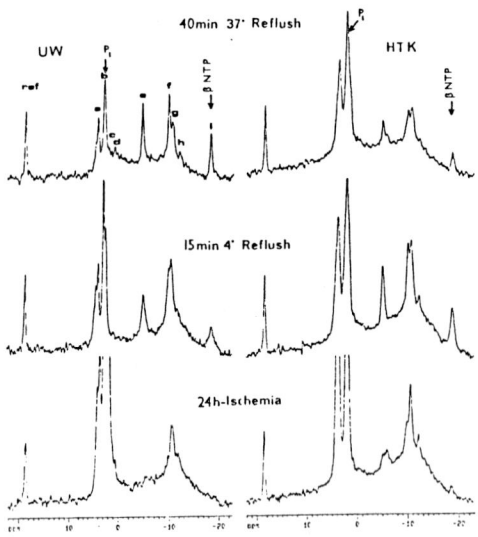

Fig 2. P-31 NMR spectra of the isolated rat liver during the sequence : 24 h cold ischemia - cold reperfusion - warm reperfusion.
Typical spectra, recorded in the course of the experiment described in the text, were selected according to the following conditions: 24 h ischemia at 4°C, reperfusion with Krebs medium at 4°C for 15 min and at 37°C for 40 min. During cold ischemia, livers were preserved in UW or HTK solution. Major resonances were assigned to (a) phophomonoesters, (b) inorganic phosphate (Pi), (c) glycerol-3 phosphorylethanolamine, (d) glycerol-3 phosphorylcholine, (e) nucleoside 5'-triphosphates (NTPg), and -diphosphates (NDPb), (f) NTPa and NDPa, (g) nicotinamide adenine dinucleotide (NAD & NADH), (h) uridine 5'-diphosphoglucose, (i) NTPb. MDPA: chemical shift reference at 18.40 ppm.

The decrease in NTP content, and the absence of pH acidosis during warm reperfusion, may be the reflection of modifications in energetic metabolism rather than irreversible injury to parenchymal cell function. As far as ATP and pHin recovery is concerned, it is necessary to prolong warm reperfusion in order to demonstrate the superiority of UW over other solutions. Our results clearly demonstrate the protecting properties of HTK solution.

To summarize, our data suggest that (a) brief cold reperfusion can restore pHin and ATP levels, (b) NTP recovery is a necessary but insufficient indicator of liver viability, (c) rates of NTP depletion and pHin decrease during cold storage depend very much on the nature of the conservation solution and could both be considered better indicators for assessing liver injury than post-ischemic NTP recovery.

II - Reperfusion injury

The ultra-simplified scheme of reperfusion injury (Parks, Granger 1988) presented in table 5 illustrates that damage occurs primarily during reperfusion and not during storage (Caldwell-Kenkel 1991). Numerous experiments have been attempted to elucidate the exact causes of injury and to propose drugs that can prevent this cascade of related events. Since the site of action of drugs or solutions is probably however multicellular and multifactorial it is difficult to propose any significant classification. There are nonetheless drugs that are primarily antioxidants (table 6), others that act on the microcirculation such as anti PAF (Ontell et al 1988), prostaglandins, calcium channel blockers (Takei 1990), papave-

Table 5. Reperfusion injury: hypothesis

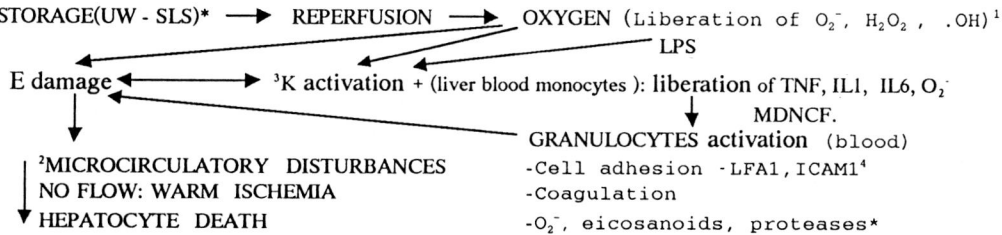

*Proteases inhibitors : leupeptine, pepstatine A, phenylmethylsulfonide fluoride diisopropyl fluorophosphate, aprotinin
SLS : sodium lactobionate sucrose solution (simplified but improved UW solution)
1: See Table 6, 2 :see Table 7, 3: see Table 8, 4: see Table 10

Table 6. Prevention of reperfusion injury by drugs (box)

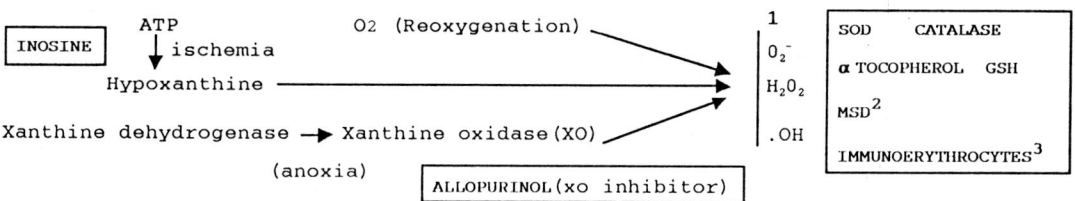

[1] Cells involved: - Hepatocytes ? - Kupffer cells - Granulocytes - Endothelial cells (contain XO) [2] Membrane stabilizing drugs (i.e. CPZ) [3] Erythrocytes contain a high level of endogenous antioxidants (Rao et al 1990)

Table 7. Carolina rinse: composition

NaCl 115 mM   KCl 5 mM   CaCL2 1.3 mM
KH2 PO4 1 mM   Mg SO4 1.2 mM

Hydroxyethyl starch (oncontic support)
Allopurinol 1 mM - Desferrioxamine 1 mM - Glutathione 3 mM (antioxidants against oxygen-based free radicals)
Fructose - Glucose - Insuline 100 u/l (Substrates to generate ATP)
Nicardipine 2 µM - Adenosine 1 µM (Vasodilators)

Table 8. Evidence for Kupffer cell activation during preservation injury

- Morphological activation
- Protease inhibitors: ↗ survival
- Nisoldipine (calcium channel blockers): ↘ survival, ↘ carbon uptake
- Carolina rinse: Prevention of reperfusion injury, ↗ survival

rine and pentoxifylline (Chazouillères et al 1988). Carolina rinse (table 7) a solution with a normal electrolytic balance, has been proposed as a cold solution to flush UW solution and provide the necessary components to prevent reperfusion injury. It is thought that Carolina rinse could prevent Kupffer cell activation (table 8).

III - MORPHOLOGY OF SINUSOIDAL CELLS DURING PRESERVATION

The weight of UW-stored livers remains virtually stable (-7.9% after 48 h of storage); hepatocytes show no significant change in surface area after 24 h storage and there is almost no ultrastructural damage, even after 48 h storage. These results definitively establish the superiority of UW over EC cold solution which induces liver swelling (+ 29.7 % after 48 h storage), enlargement of mean hepatocyte area (+ 24.3% after 24 h storage) with swollen and degenerated hepatocytes (after 48 h storage). The large molecular compounds, lactobionate and raffinose, present in UW, as against the glucose in EC, are thought to prevent water influx to cells.
Microvascular injury is one of the chief causes of preservation failure after prolonged storage (McKeown et al 1988, Momii et al 1990, Caldwell- Kenkel et al 1991). So far only one group has differentiated changes occurring during storage from changes occurring during storage plus reperfusion, but even in this case the experiment was carried out with Krebs Ringer solution. No whole blood or OLT experiments have yet been reported. According to Caldwell- Kenkel et al 1991 there are two stages in storage injury -1- the potentially reversible damage that occurs during cold ischemia storage and makes the tissue susceptible to lethal reperfusion injury, and -2- reperfusion injury itself (table 9). Lethal injury occurs to endothelial cells after brief reperfusion and prohibits graft success. Microcirculatory disturbances as shown by video fluorescence microscopy are greater in transplanted livers that have been previously stored under survival rather than in non-survival conditions. Activated Kupffer cells release soluble toxic mediators than can contribute to microcirculatory dysfunction. Kupffer cell activation could occur in response to factors released by injured endothelial cells.

IV - INTERPLAY BETWEEN DONOR, PRESERVATION AND REJECTION

It is becoming clear that in humans, preservation injury may predispose to rejection (Howard et al 1990, Campbell et al 1991). In 215 cases of consecutive OLT, on arrival in the intensive care unit, 70 patients were thought to have severe preservation injury (ASAT > 2000 IU/L) and 35 moderate preservation injury (ASAT <600 IU/L). In the first group 12% had no rejection, 71% had rejection and 18% had graft loss versus 64, 33 and 3% in the second. There was no difference in the severity of rejection between the 2 groups. Damage to or necrosis of endothelial cells and parenchymal cells, plus activation of Kupffer cells, could attract inflammatory cells (lymphocytes, macrophages) and as a result increase the expression of major histocompatibility complex and adhesion molecules (table 10) (Burke

Table 9 : Sequence of morphological changes occurring during liver preservation.

Eurocollins: Rat liver[1]
  S:4-8 h
a) **Endothelial cells.** S: retraction of many cytoplasmic extensions : sinusoidal lining formed of strands of coalesced beads of cytoplasm. S + R : in some areas the lining is normal (return of the lining to a more extended configuration); in others, cells are beginning to lose their viability : fusion of clusters of small fenestrations into large openings - retraction of cytoplasmic processes forming thick strands - rounding of the perinuclear cytoplasm
b) **Kupffer cells.** S: normal. S + R : some vacuolisation and formation of granules
c) **Hepatocytes.** S: swollen - hepatocellular blebs projecting into the sinusoidal lumen. S + R: well preserved.
  S:16-24 h
a) **Endothelial cells.** S: the structure is obscured by sinusoidal blebs - cytoplasmic retraction is more severe than after 8 h storage - plasma membranes appear intact - mitochondria are frequently swollen. S + R : complete loss of cell viability - destruction of the sinusoidal lining (denudation) - rounded, spherical nuclear regions projecting into the sinusoidal lumen - shredded, string-shaped cytoplasmic processes.
b) **Kupffer cells.** S : some rounding cells with occasional short ruffles on their surfaces. S + R : signs of activation : increased volume - surface composed of complex folds and extensions (filopodia - lamellipodia) - deep slitlike invaginations of the plasma membrane - vacuolization of the cytoplasm and formation of granules within vacuoles polarized toward the luminal surface - release of acid phosphatase
c) **Hepatocytes.** S: hepatocellular swelling and blebbing (more severe in the periportal region). S + R : shrinkage of some cells due to bleb shedding - rapid disappearance of blebs (shedding and resorption).

UNIVERSITY OF WISCONSIN: Rat liver [1]
  S:8 h
a) **Endothelial cells.** S: changes are less severe. S + R: better preservation of the endothelial wall
b) **Kupffer cells.** S + R: little activation
  S:16 h
a) **Endothelial cell.** S + R : most cells have not desquamated or lost viability - some appear to be able to flatten and reextend their processes.
b) **Kupffer cells.** S + R : some are activated, some relatively unchanged - less release of acid phosphatase
c) **Hepatocytes.** S : hepatocellular blebbing and swelling is greatly reduced.

UNIVERSITY O WISCONSIN: Human liver [2]
  S <12 h (in vivo situation) - Fig. 3a
S + R: adhesion of platelets and granulocytes to the endothelial wall. Kupffer cells rounded, loaded with large vacuoles. Sinusoids generally well preserved. A few, however, are damaged
  S:28 h (surgical biopsy from patients operated for tumors) - Fig. 3b
a) **Endothelial cells.** S : enlargement of fenestrae. S + R: well preserved endothelial lining - fenestrae of normal size
b) **Kupffer cells.** S : loss of pseudopodia and filipodia - rounded with blunted ruffling of the surface. S + R : similar aspect with more vacuoles
c) **Hepatocytes.** S : hepatocellular blebs in the sinusoidal lumen. S + R : a few bleb remnants in the lumen.

S: storage - **R** : Reperfusion (37°C + O2) with Krebs (rat) or RPMI (human surgical biopsy)
[1] - Caldwell - Kenkel et al 1991, [2] - Bioulac-Sage et al. in preparation

Table 10. Human HLA, AB Ag and adhesion molecules in the liver

	HLA		AB
CELLS	Class I (A, B)	Class II (DP, DQ, DR)	
Hepatocytes	± [+]	-	-
Bile duct	+++	- [++]	+
Art/venous E	++	- [+]	+++
Capillary E	++	- (DP, DQ) [+] ++ (DR)	++
Dendritic cells	+	+ (DP, DQ) ++ (DR)	-
Sinusoidal cells	+		
E		++	+
K		± (DQ) [++]	+
		++	

Expression of MHC Ag by cells is a dynamic process, influenced by many factors. [changes after OLT]

Sinusoidal endothelial adhesion molecules

	NORMAL	AFTER OLT
ICAM-1		
Hepatocytes	-	-
bile ducts	-	-
Sinusoidal cells		
endothelial	+	+/++
Kupffer	+	+/++
Intersticial cells	+	+

Endothelial cells actively modulate their surface phenotype in response to environmental factors.(Steinhoff 1990).

VLA adhesion molecules (Very Late Activation Ag)

- Cellular adhesion mechanisms (cell/cell; cell/matrix interactions) are a fundamental process in the immunobiology of the liver.
- Interactions with various ECM components are mediated by the VLA, subgroup of the INTEGRIN superfamily of adhesion molecules.
- 6 different VLA dimers:
  .serve as receptors for ECM components : laminin (VLA-1,3,6) - Co(VLA-1,2,3) - fibronectin (VLA-4,5)
  .function as homing receptors for leucocytes (VLA-4)

* Expression of VLA-4 homing receptor on sinusoidal lining cells in inflammatory liver disease may favor the recruitment of VLA - 4 + leucocytes in liver parenchyma.

et al 1991), thus rendering the liver more susceptible to rejection (Kurozumi et al 1991). In addition purified hepatocytes can stimulate T lymphocytes.

It is also possible to modulate Kupffer cell activity in the donor, and either improve the chances of graft survival by injecting latex particles 24 h prior to preservation or prevent parenchymal cell damage induced by 24 h hypothermic preservation by feeding rats a diet deficient in essential fatty acid for 2.5 months, a regimen known to deplete tissues of arachidonic acid and to inhibit several macrophage functions including the synthesis of eicosanoids.

It is also known that the nutritional status of the donor plays an important role in rat liver preservation (i.e.in the isolated rat liver perfusion model, total parenteral nutrition versus isotonic dextrose infusion improves metabolic condition, portal hemodynamics and prevents hepatic injury). FK506, the new immunosuppressive drug, has also been shown to have a protective effect against hepatic ischemia (Sakr 1991).

CONCLUSION

Human OLT can safely be performed after 12 h preservation in UW cold solution (D'Allessandro et al 1990) and this period can probably be extended to 24 h (Furukawa et al 1991). Beyond 36-48 h it becomes difficult to perfuse the liver because of extensive sinusoidal and also hepatocytic damage.
In animal studies, this period has been extented with the use of the machine perfusion in the dog (preservation time of 72 h).
To-day the mechanisms involved, that have made this progress possible, are still unknown, but it can be speculated that the continuous flushing of sinusoids represents a major factor.It is likely that similar results may soon be obtained for human liver, which could make it possible even to envisage the setting-up of a short- term liver bank. The liver, both in terms of cells and functions, is an heterogeneous organ and preservation can only be a compromise reconciling diverse requirements.It is probably necessary to study preservation procedures firstly cell by cell,and then by successive cell combination (with the appropriate cell matrix)

in order to understand these different, and no doubt, often opposing requirements. Liver preservation is still in its early days.

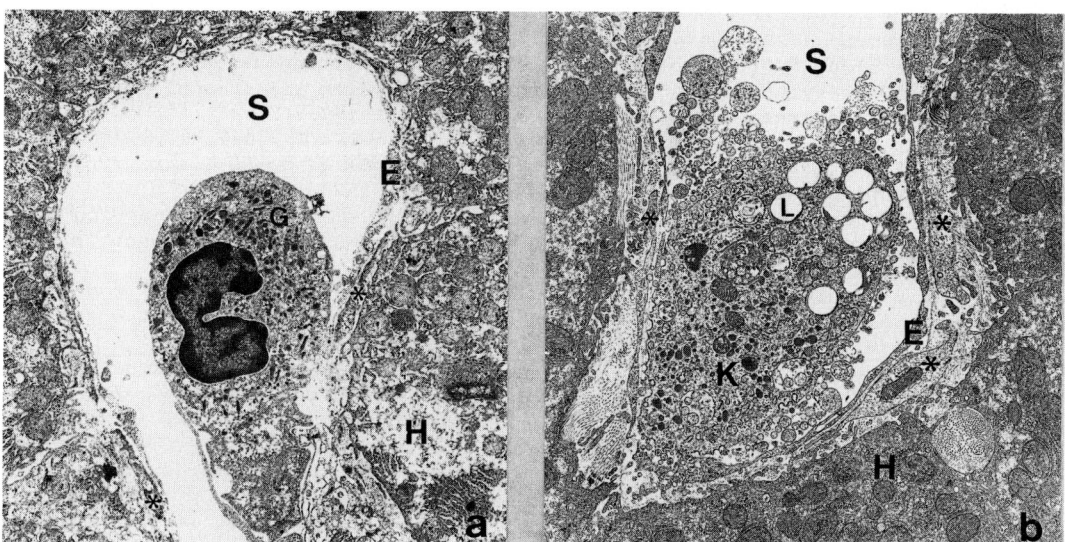

Fig.3 -a- human liver. Preservation in UW (12 h), revascularisation (2 h): relatively well-preserved endothelial wall. Adhesion of a granulocyte (G) to the endothelial wall (E) x 4,500. -b- human liver. Biopsy preserved 28 h in UW. Reperfusion with RPMI: good preservation of sinusoidal cells, rounded and active Kuffer cell (with latex particles L) x 6,200.
H: hepatocyte; S: sinusoidal lumen; asterisk: perisinusoidal process

AKNOWLEDGEMENTS

This work was supported by grants from the Conseil Régional d'Aquitaine

REFERENCES

Belzer, F.O., Southard, J.H. (1988) : Principles of solid-organ preservation by cold storage. Transplantation 45 : 673-676.
Burke, E.C., Martinez, O.M., Freise, C.E., McVicar, Roberts, J.P., Ascher, N.L. (1991) : MHC expression on human hepatocytes before and after isolation. Transplant. Proc. 23 : 1428-1429.
Caldwell-Kenkel, J.C., Currin, R.T., Tanaka, Y., Thurman, R.G., Lemasters, J.J. (1989) : Reperfusion injury to endothelial cells following cold ischemic storage of rat livers. Hepatology 10 : 292-299.
Caldwell-Kenkel, J.C., Currin, R.T., Tanaka, Y., Thurman, R.G., Lemasters, J.J. (1991) : Kuffer cell activation and endothelial cell damage after storage of rat livers : effects of reperfusion. Hepatology 13 : 83-95
Campbell, D.A., Merion, R.M., Ham, J.M., Lucey, M.R., Henley, K.S., Turcotte, G. (1991) : Hepatic preservation with university of Wisconsin solution is associated with reduced allograft rejection. Transplant. Proc. 23 : 1547-1549.
Chazouillères, O., Ballet, F., Chrétien, Y., Marteau, P., Rey, C., Maillard, D., Poupon, R. (1989) : Protective effect of vasodilators on liver function after long hypothermic preservation : a study in the isolated perfused rat liver. Hepatology 9 : 824-829.

D'Alessandro, A.M., Kalayoglu, M., Sollinger, H.W., Hoffmann, R.M., Pirsch, J.D., Lorentzen, D.F., Melzer, J.S., Belzer, F.O. (1990) : Experience with Belzer UW cold storage solution in human liver transplantation. Transplant. Proc. 22 : 474-476.

Desmoulin F, Cozzone PJ, Canioni P.(1987): Phosphorus-31 Nuclear Magnetic Resonance study of phosphorylated metabolites compartmentation, intracellular pH and phosphorylation state during normoxia, hypoxia and ethanol perfusion, in the perfused rat liver. Eur J Biochem 162, 151-159.

Furukawa, H., Todo, S., Imventarza, O., Wu, Y.M., Scotti, C., Day, R., Starzl, T.E. (1991) : Cold ischemia time vs outcome of human liver transplantation using UW solution. Transplant. Proc. 23 : 1550-1551.

Holzmueller P, Reckendorfer H, Burgmann H, Moser E.(1990): Viability testing of transplantation donor liver by 1H NMR relaxometry. Magnetic Resonance in Medicine 16, 173-181.

Howard, T.K., Klintmalm, G.B.G., Cofer, J.B., Husberg, B.S., Goldstein, R.M., Gonwa, T.A. (1990) : The influence of preservation injury on rejection in the hepatic transplant recipient. Transplantation 49 : 103-107.

Howden BO, Jablonsky P, Thomas AC, Walls K, Biguzas M, Scott DF, Grossman H, Marshall VC.(1990): Liver preservation with UW solution. Evidence that hydroxyethyl starch is not essential. Transplantation 49, 869-872.

Kurozumi, Y., Sakagami, K., Orita, K. (1991) : Ex vivo perfusion of the liver with anti-class II antibody can prevent acute rejection in canine liver transplantation. Transplant. Proc. 23 : 593-596.

McKeown, C.M.B., Edwards, V., Phillips, M.J., Harvey, P.R.C., Petrunka, C.N., Strasberg, S.M. (1988) : Sinusoidal lining cell damage : the critical injury in cold preservation of liver allografts in the rat. Transplantation 46 : 178-191.

Momii, S., Koga, A. (1990) : Time-related morphological changes in cold-stored rat livers. Transplantation 50 : 745-750.

Ontell, S.J., Makowka, L., Ove, P., Starzl, T.E. (1988) : Improved hepatic function in the 24-hour preserved rat liver with UW-lactobionate solution and SRI 63-411. Gastroenterology 95 : 1617-1624.

Parks, D.A., Granger, D.N. (1988) : Ischelia-reperfusion injury : a radical view. Hepatology 8 : 680-682.

Pienaar, B.H., Lindell, S.L., Vaan Gulik, T., Southard, J.H., Belzer, F.O. (1990): Seventy-two-hour preservation of the canine liver by machine perfusion.Transplantation 49 : 258-260.

Rao, P.N., Walsh, T.R., Makowka, L., Liu, T., Demetris, A.J., Rubin, R.S., Snyder, J.T., Mischinger, H.J., Starzl, T.E. (1990) : Inhibition of free radical generation and improved survival by protection of the hepatic microvascular endothelium by targeted erythrocytes in orthotopic rat liver transplantation. Transplantation 49 : 1055-1059.

Sakr, M.F., Zetti, G.M., Farghali, H., Hassanein, T.H., Gavaler, J.S., Starzl, T.E., Van Thiel, D. H. (1991) : Protective effect of FK 506 against hepatic ischemia in rats. Transplant. Proc. 23 : 340-341.

Southard, J.H., Van Gulik, T.M., Amenati, M.S., Vreugdenhil, P.K., Lindell, S.L., Pienaar, B.L., Belzer, F.O. (1990) : Important components of the UW solution. Transplantation 49 : 251-257

Steinhoff, G., Behrend, M., Pichlmayr, R. (1990) : Induction of ICAM-1 on Hepatocyte membranes during liver allograft rejection and infection. Transplant. Proc. 22 : 2308-2309.

Takei, Y., Marzi, I., Kauffman, F.C., Currin, R.T., Lemasters, J.J., Thurman, R.G. (1990) : Increase in survival time of liver transplants by protease inhibitors and a calcium channel blocker, nisoldipine. Transplantation 50 : 14-20

Liver transplantation - Immunological aspects of preservation and liver function

Gustav Steinhoff

Klinik für Abdominal und Transplantations-chirurgie, Medizinische Hochschule Hannover, PO Box 610180, D-3000 Hannover 61, Germany

Liver inflammation represents a wide range of immune events occuring after liver transplantation. These are associated with immunological changes of donor graft cells and different states of immune reactivity of infiltrating host leucocytes. The rejection response to histoincompatible major histocompatibility complex (MHC, HLA-system) and non-MHC antigens forms the natural cause of specific organ damage. However, nonspecific inflammation occurs in other pathological situations as with preservation injury, bacterial/viral infection and toxic damage of the liver. Immune reactions in the graft are accompagnied by immunological changes on graft cells as portal and sinusoidal endothelia, Kupffer cells, bile ducts, and hepatocytes. Major changes occur in the expression of immune adhesion molecules (ICAM-1, LFA-3, ELAM-1, VCAM-1) and MHC class I (HLA-A,B,C) and class II (HLA-DR,DP,DQ) antigens that are upregulated with inflammation together with the release of cytokines. The cellular infiltration by recipient leucocytes during immune reactions leads to a partial or total exchange of donor antigen presenting accessory cells (Kupffer cells, portal dendritic cells). This loss of immune competent donor accessory cells may cause an altered presentation of donor MHC-antigens and influence immune reactivity to the graft. Changes in the inflammatory state and cellular composition of the liver graft may influence liver function and the course of rejection and infections after transplantation.

IMMUNE REACTIONS AFTER LIVER TRANSPLANTATION

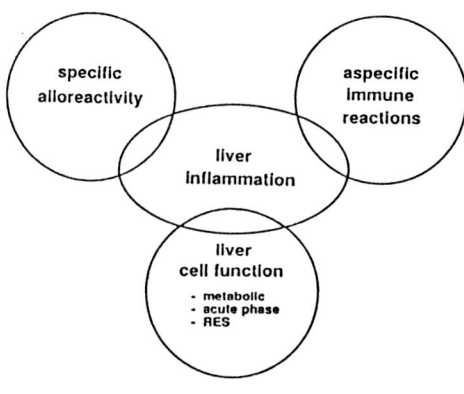

Immunological functions of the grafted liver

Beside metabolic functions a number of immunological functions are exerted by liver cells. So far known these include especially the processing and presentation of microbial particles and antigens by Kupffer cells. Furthermore, passing leucocytes and lymphocytes can be activated by direct cellular contact to sinusoidal cells mediated by adhesion molecules, MHC, cytokines and complement factors (Hogg, 1989; Springer, 1990; Unanue, 1987; Mantovani, 1989). In addition, the production of cytokines as interleukins, interferons, eicanosoids and growth factors (GM-CSF) by liver endothelia, Kupffer cells and hepatocytes may influence bone marrow and leucocyte reactivity systemically by the blood stream. In this context also the production of soluble MHC-molecules and beta-2 microglobulin by liver cells during inflammatory reactions can be regarded as a systemical reaction (Ramadori et al, 1989; Davies et al, 1989). These reactions probably form part of many different systemical immune reactions particularly during severe infections.

It is assumable that in the liver transplant immune functions are impaired in a similar way as metabolical in situations of preservation damage and during inflammatory reactions as rejection. The question arises, which changes occur in the molecular expression of immune receptor/ligand molecules and cytokine production as the cellular composition of the graft. Changes in the inflammatory state of the graft itself can modulate the immune reactivity of the host by altering the expression of adhesion molecules and release of cytokines. Moreover, the transplant situation with partial MHC (HLA)-incompatibility may interfere with cell functions that include those by MHC-receptor molecules. Incompatibility of class II MHC-antigens may then lead to decreased or non-reactivity of CD-4+ T-helper lymphocytes to microbial and viral antigen presenting (accessory) cells as Kupffer cells, portal dendritic cells and endothelia. In addition, the effects of alloreactivity of a major number of helper T-cell clones may impair normal immune reactivity to viral and microbial in the transplanted liver. On the other hand, the production of soluble (allo) class I MHC-molecules by liver cells after transplantation may interfere with alloreactivity to these antigens and influence immune reactivity up to a state of specific tolerance (Davies et al, 1989).

Immunological functions of the liver

Endothelial cells
 - antigen presentation
 - lymphocyte/leucocyte homing
   and activation
 - cytokine production

Kupffer cells
 - phagocytosis
 - antigen presentation
 - cytokine production

Hepatocytes
 - acute phase: cytokines/soluble MHC

Portal interstitial dendritic cells
 - antigen presentation
 - lymphocyte stimulation
 - cytokine production

Immune sequelae of preservation injury

The process of organ cooling in the donor and the cold and warm ischemia time up to revascularization in the recipient involves a varying degree of organ damage. Many studies have clearly shown the metabolic changes leading to impaired organ function after preservation injury. Especially ultrastructural studies by the group of Bioulac-Sage/Balabaud and McKeown (1989) have demonstrated damage of sinusoidal endothelia and activation of Kupffer cells corresponding to degrees of organ damage by ischemia and perfusion. A major contribution to the preservation injury makes the reperfusion damage of infiltrating leucocytes of the host in the first hours after transplantation (Thurmann et al, 1988). Shackleton et al (1990) have demonstrated in an experimental rat liver transplantation model that class I and class II MHC-molecules were induced in the graft after recovery from ischemic injury. It has to be assumed that the activation of graft endothelia and Kupffer cells may induce the recruitment and infiltration of leucocytes. A major pathway of this reaction is probably the induction of adhesion molecules on graft cells before and during transplantation (Steinhoff et al, 1990) as the release of cytokines. It is possible, that the process of liver inflammation is further propagated with reduced function of the liver RES as a result of preservation injury. This may lead to endotoxemia and septic problems, but on the other hand also induce leucocyte preactivation in the blood stream. A temporary loss of functions of sinusoidal endothelia and Kupffer cells and a lesser clearance of microbial antigens as endotoxins may be the result of preservation injury in the liver. A further sequelae of liver inflammation caused by preservation injury may be the induction of a rejection response. Howard et al (1990) have reported a higher incidence of severe rejection episodes in initially bad functioning graft. It is likely that graft inflammation causing the induction of donor MHC-antigens and recruitment of alloreactive lymphocytes may be enhanced in the early postoperative period despite strong immunosuppression.

Preservation injury after liver transplantation

---

1. aspecific liver inflammation
   - activation of endothelia, Kupffer cells, hepatocytes
   - recruitment and infiltration of leucocytes

2. reduced immunological function of the liver (RES)

3. induction of alloantigens (MHC) and rejection (?)

Immunological changes in the donor liver before and directly after transplantation

In own studies (Steinhoff et al, 1988, 1989, 1990) and by other authors (Daar et al, 1984) a number of immunological changes have been observed in biopsies of donor organs and during liver transplantation. Firstly, the expression of class I and class II MHC-antigens of the donor is altered in most grafts. Class I (HLA-A,B,C) antigens are increased expressed on donor hepatocytes even in biopsies taken before transplantation. Also the expression of class II (HLA-DR) antigens on sinusoidal endothelia was elevated in these grafts. Recently, we also could find a simultaneous induction of immune adhesion molecules. Table 1 gives a summary of these findings. Especially the expression of ICAM-1, LFA-3 and VCAM-1 on sinusoidal endothelia was elevated in most graft biopsies studied at the time of transplantation.

Table 1

Induction of immune adhesion molecules and major histocompatibility antigens (MHC) during liver transplantation*

Immune adhesion molecules

ICAM-1,LFA-3,VCAM-1:
- induced on sinusoidal endothelia, Kupffer cells
- unchanged on hepatocytes, bile duct, portal and centralvenous endothelia

MHC-molecules

class I (HLA-A,B):
- induced on hepatocytes, bile duct epithelia

class II (HLA-DR,DP)
- induced on sinusoidal endothelia, (ev. bile duct epithelia)

---

* Comparison of biopsies of normal resected liver (n=7) and biopsies taken before and during transplantation (n=30)

A second observation in donor and intraoperative biopsies was an increased infiltration of the sinusoids by leucocytes. Immunohistological staining with monoclonal antibodies to donor or recipient HLA-antigens (Steinhoff et al, 1987) revealed that the vast majority of these cells were of donor type. So far analysis of the cells with lineage specific monoclonal antibodies (reacting with monocytes, granulocytes or lymphocytes) revealed that the majority of the cells were immature monocytes/granulocytes of donor type (double staining with donor HLA) (Steinhoff et al, 1989). These cells most likely have just immigrated in the hours or days before transplantation in the donor. At the same time, the population of mature Kupffer cells was decreased in most biopsies. As inflammatory reactions after transplantation also induce an exchange of Kupffer cells corresponding to the infiltration of immature monocytes differentiating to Kupffer cells (Steinhoff et al, 1989) this also has to be assumed for the disease situation of the donor before transplantation. In addition to monocytes and granulocytes a high number of donor lymphocytes are transplanted

Immunological changes in the donor liver before and directly after transplantation

---

1. Endothelial damage and activation
    - induction of class II MHC-antigens (donor)
    - induction of adhesion molecules (ICAM-1)
    - cytokine release (?)
    - complement (?)

2. Leucocyte infiltration of the sinusoids
    - increased numbers of 27E10+ monocytes/granulocytes
    - increased numbers of donor lymphocytes

3. Kupffer cell activation and exchange
    - increased numbers of immature donor Kupffer cells
    - reduced numbers of mature Kupffer cells (days)
    - induction of donor class I and class II MHC, adhesion molecules (LFA-1,ICAM-1)

4. MHC class I expression by hepatocytes and bile ducts

---

with the graft (Schlitt, Kanehiro, Steinhoff et al, unpublished). At the present time the immunological effects of these cells (graft versus host activity) are under investigation.

Immunological factors affecting early graft function

The analysis of graft biopsies during transplantation revealed a number of changes indicating immune activation and inflammation of sinusoidal cells either in the donor or shortly after reperfusion. Secondly the transplant procedure including cold perfusion, ischemia and sudden revascularisation is a major insult to the metabolic function of liver cells leading to temporal dysfunction and partial cell death. This induces a second phase of immune activation in the graft and subsequent leucocyte recruitment in the hours and days after transplantation. This may be beneficial to repair processes, but also affect the graft integrity by further inflammatory reactions. Especially injury to sinusoidal endothelia and microvascular stasis (infiltration/cytokine release) may affect the vascularisation of the parenchyma and result in further organ damage.

A third factor to enface is the primary immune response to the allograft. Although - especially with strong perioperative immunosuppression - the lymphocyte response may be very limited, specific anti-alloantigenic reactions may be initiated by antibodies to blood group antigens (ABO and minor blood groups) and preformed antibodies to HLA-antigens (at retransplantation, after blood transfusion). Ultimately this can lead to a humoral type of rejection (Demetris et al,1989).

Inflammation of the liver shortly after transplantation either caused by preservation injury, postoperative leucocyte infiltration or "hyperacute" humoral rejection may affect the capacity of the liver to clear microbial antigens and endotoxins. So far no clinical studies have been able to measure the function of the RES in these situations. The factors mentioned above, however, in addition to the immunosuppression given are likely to exert major temporal changes in the immunological integrity of the transplanted liver.

Immunological factors affecting early graft function
___

1. endothelial damage and activation
2. leucocyte mediated tissue injury
3. antibody mediated ("hyperacute") rejection
4. Kupffer cell dysfunction (?)
___

Inflammation of the transplanted liver

The immunological factors impairing liver function in the early postoperative period also may play an important role in the genesis of late dysfunction. Of course, the allograft rejection response forms the cause of specific organ damage. Interestingly, however, lymphocyte reactivity is mainly restricted to the portal tract (portal endothelia, bile ducts, portal insterstitial infiltration). Parenchymal infiltration and periportal necrosis is a rather advanced event in the rejection process. The rejection response, however, is not a singular lymphocyte effector process, but involves many other unspecific leucocyte reactions. Moreover, it could be demonstrated, that sinusoidal cells (endothelia and Kupffer cells) as hepatocytes and bile ducts are induced to express additional adhesion ligand molecules during liver inflammation (Adams et al, 1989; Steinhoff et al, 1990). Especially the induction of ICAM-1 and LFA-3 could be noted with rejection and non-rejection related inflammation. This process is most likely a potent regulator of LFA-1+ leucocyte adhesion and activation (Springer, 1990; Krensky et al, 1990). Moreover, the broad induction of MHC class I and class II (Steinhoff, 1990) as adhesion molecules in the parenchyma is an indicator of the local and systemic increase of cytokines (IL-1, gamma Interferon) (Dustin et al,1986 and 1988; Springer 1990). In our group Hoffmann et al (1991) could demonstrate elevated cytokine levels (IL-1, TNF) in liver graft biopsies during rejection and infection.

The inflammatory reaction in the graft thus alters its exposition and secretion of immune regulatory molecules. This recruits and stimulates leucocytes and mediates their infiltration. Interestingly, there is a predilection of infiltrates for the portal tract and central vein region. In the sinusoids, however, no local infiltration is common. The cellular content of the sinusoids, however, is increased and Kupffer cells are activated. The ongoing sinusoidal inflammation during rejection and infection then leads to a gradual or rapid loss of mature Kupffer cells and infiltration/replacement by monocytes (Steinhoff et al, 1987 and 1989; Gouw et al, 1987; Gassel et al, 1987). Similarly to the situation occuring after preservation and organ transplantation a temporal decrease in RES-capacity can be postulated during severe liver inflammation. This may be one cause for septic and toxic complications in the course of liver transplant rejection.

Specific immunosuppression as with cyclosporin A or FK506 affects T-lymphocyte reactivity and cytokine release, but may leave the unspecific liver inflammation partly unaffected. It is very well possible that the process of parenchymal activation and subsequent inflammation may escape immunosuppression and itself generate chronic stimulation by the additional induction of donor MHC-antigens. Humoral effector mechanisms and intercurrent viral infection may also play part in the generation of treatment resistant rejection types.

Inflammation of liver transplants
during infection and rejection
___

- cytokine production / systemic reaction
- impaired liver function (RES),
  septic complications
- escape of immunosuppression
- additional induction and sensitization
  to alloantigens
- additional induction of adhesion molecules
  and recruitment of leucocytes (CSF)

___

Changes in the cellular and molecular composition of the graft - longterm adaptation

The question arises, if changes in the molecular and cellular composition of the graft, that occur during and in the course after transplantation, have an effect on the longterm immunological adaptation. It has become clear, that the regulation of immune regulatory molecules as MHC-products, adhesion molecule ligands, cytokines and complement underlies major changes during minor and major complications. As a result of inflammation, however, a major part of the grafts immunocompetent cells (Kupffer cells, portal interstitial dendritic cells) is exchanged (Gale et al; 1978; Steinhoff et al, 1987,1989; Gouw et al, 1987; Austyn et al, 1990; Prickett et al, 1988). This leads to a lesser basic expression of alloantigens in the late course after transplantation. In addition, immunosuppression probably reduces the stimulatory signals leading to upregulation of inflammatory reactions. This may leave the graft less susceptible to the immune assault at late term after transplantation and explain the clinical experience of a good longterm graft function. It is not excluded, however, that intercurrent infection and toxic damage induces liver inflammation and generates a secondary antiallogenic immune response at late term.

REFERENCES

Adams, D. H., S. G. Hubscher, J. Shaw, R. Rothlein, J. M. Neuberger. Intercellular adhesion molecule 1 on liver allografts during rejection. Lancet 1989: 1122 - 1125

Austyn J.M., C.P. Larsen. Migration patterns of dendritic leukocytes: implications for transplantation. Transplantation 1990;49:1-7.

Daar, A. S., S. V. Fuggle, J. W. Fabre, A. Ting, P. J. Morris. The detailed distribution of HLA-A,B,C antigens in normal human organs. Transplantation 1984; 38: 287 - 292

Davies HffS., Pollard S.G., Calne R.Y. Soluble HLA-antigens in the circulation of liver graft recipients. Transplantation 1989;47:524-527.

Demetris AJ, Jaffe R, Tzakis A et al. Antibody mediated rejection of human orthotopic liver allografts. A J Pathol 1988; 132:489.

Dustin, M.L., R. Rothlein, A.K. Bhan, C.A. Dinarello, T.A. Springer. Induction by IL 1 and Interferon-g: Tissue distribution, biochemistry, and function of a natural adherence molecule (ICAM-1). J Immunol 1986; 137: 245 - 254

Dustin, M.L., D.E. Staunton, T.A. Springer. Supergene families meet in the immune system. Immunol Today 1988; 9: 213 - 215

Gale, R.P., R. S. Sparkes, D. W. Golde. Bone marrow origin of hepatic macrophages (Kupffer cells) in humans. Science 1978; 201: 937 - 938

Gassel, H. J., R. Engemann, A. Thiede, H. Hamelmann. Replacement of donor Kupffer cells by recipient cells after orthotopic rat liver transplantation. Transplant Proc 1987; 19: 351 - 353

Gouw, A. S. H., H. J. Houthoff, S. Huitema, J. M. Beelen, C. H. Gips, S. Poppema. Expression of major histocompatibility complex antigens and replacement of donor cells by recipient ones in human liver grafts. Transplantation 1987; 43: 291 - 296

Hoffmann, M. W., Wonigeit, K., Steinhoff, G., Behrend, M., Herzbeck, H., Flad, H.-D., Pichlmayr, R. Tumor necrosis factor alpha and interleukin-1 beta in rejecting human liver grafts. Transplant Proc in Druck

Hogg, N. The leukocyte integrins. Immunol Today 1989; 10: 111 - 114

Howard T.K., Klintmalm G.B.G., Cofer J.B., Husberg B.S., Goldstein R.N., Gouwa T.A. The influence of preservation injury on rejection in the hepatic transplant recipient. Transplantation 1990;49:103-106.

Krensky, A. M., A. Weiss, G. Crabtree, M. M. Davis, P. Parham. T-Lymphocyte-Antigen Interactions in Transplant Rejection. New Engl J Med 1990; 322: 510 - 517

Mantovani, A., E. Dejana. Cytokines as communication signals between leukocytes and endothelial cells. Immunol Today 1989; 10: 370 - 375

McKeown C.M.B., V. Edwards, M.J. Philipps. P.R.C. Marvey, C.N. Perunha, S.M. Strasberg. Sinusoidal lining cell damage: The critical injury in cold preservation of liver allografts in the rat. Transplantation 1989;46:178-191.

Prickett, T.C.R., J.L. McKenzie, D.N.J. Hart. Characterization of interstitial dendritic cells in human liver. Transplantation 1988; 46: 754 - 761

Ramadori G., A. Mitsch, H. Rieder, K.H. Meyer zum Büschenfelde. Alpha- and gamma-interferon (IFN alpha, IGN gamma) but not interleukin-1 (IL-1) modulate synthesis and secretion of beta-2 microglobulin by hepatocytes. Eur J Clin Invest 1988;18:343-51.

Shackleton C.R., S.L. Ettinger, M.G. McLoughlin, C.H. Sandamore, R.R. Miller, P.A. Keown. Effect of recovery from ischemic injury on class I and class II MHC antigen expression. Transplantation 1990;49:641-644.

Springer, T. A. Adhesion receptors of the immune system. Nature 1990; 346: 425 - 434

Steinhoff G, Wonigeit K, Harpprecht J, Johnson JP, Pichlmayr R. Expression of donor and recipient class I and class II MHC-antigens in human liver grafts. Transplant Proc 1987,XIX;3761-3764.

Steinhoff G, Wonigeit K, Pichlmayr R. Analysis of sequential changes in major histocompatibility complex expression in human liver grafts after transplantation. Transplantation 1988;45:394-401.

Steinhoff G, Wonigeit K, Sorg C, Behrend M, Mues B, Pichlmayr R. Patterns of macrophage immigration and differentiation in human liver grafts. Transplant Proc 1989;21(1):398-401.

Steinhoff G, Behrend M, Sorg C, Wonigeit K, Pichlmayr R. Sequential analysis of macrophage tissue differentiation and Kupffer cell exchange after human liver transplantation. In " Cells of the Hepatic Sinusoids Vol.II" (Editors: E Wisse, DL Knook, K. Decker) Rijswijk, NL, 1989;406-409.

Steinhoff G. Major histocompatibility complex antigens in human liver grafts. J Hepatol, 1990;11:9.

Steinhoff G, Behrend M, Wonigeit K. Expression of adhesion molecules on lymphocytes/monocytes and hepatocytes in human liver grafts. Human Immunol, 1990;28:123.

Thurmann R.G., I. Marzi, G. Seitz, J. Thies, J.J. Lemasters, F. Zimmermann. Hepatic reperfusion injury following orthotopic liver transplantation in the rat. Transplantation 1988;46:502-506

Unanue, E. R., P. M. Allen. The basis for the immunoregulatory role of macrophages and other accessory cells. Science 1987; 236: 551 - 557.

The tolerance induced by liver allografting

Yvon Calmus, Didier Houssin

Laboratoire de Recherche Chirurgicale et Laboratoire d'Immunologie, Faculté de Médecine Cochin-Port-Royal, 75014 Paris, France

It is currently assumed that liver allografts are less intensively rejected than other organs. Hyperacute rejection is rare or absent in man (Iwatsuki 1981). In some rat and pig allogeneic combinations, orthotopic liver allografting leads to a state of donor-specific tolerance without immunosuppression, whereas, under the same conditions, heart and kidney allografts are usually rejected (Houssin 1980, Houssin 1983, Zimmerman 1984, Kamada 1985). Furthermore, in these experimental combinations, the presence of the tolerated liver allograft induces a state of MHC-specific systemic tolerance for all other organs or tissues of the same donor (Houssin 1980, Kamada 1985).

Characteristics of the immune status of liver-induced tolerance.

Analysis of the tolerance state in the recipient of a tolerated liver allograft reveals a state of "split" tolerance at both the cellular and humoral level. Indeed, spleen cells from tolerant recipient show a normal proliferative response in mixed lymphocyte culture, but fail to develop cytotoxic activity against donor target cells in cell-mediated lysis, a defect which is specific for the tolerated donor alloantigens (Kamada 1985). The fact that the cytotoxic response is suppressed while the proliferative response is preserved suggests either a selective clonal deletion of class I alloreactive T cells or the induction of specific suppressor cells (Nossal 1989). The antibody response shows a rapid disappearance of anti-MHC class I antibodies, while anti-class II antibodies remain at high levels for several months. In contrast, both anti-class I and anti-class II antibodies remain at high levels in recipients grafted with allogeneic skin (Kamada 1985).

Possible mechanisms of liver-induced tolerance.

1. Particular MHC expression.

MHC molecules play a major role in allograft rejection. MHC class II are the main inducers of the allogenic immune response, while the presence of MHC class I molecules is required for efficient lysis of target cells by cytotoxic T lymphocytes (Hansen 1989, Ascher 1987, Ferry 1987). Hepatic MHC class I expression is normally limited in the human liver to sinusoidal and biliary cells while MHC class II expression is restricted to sinusoidal and dendritic cells (Rouger 1986, Lautenschlager 1984, Franco 1988). Hepatocytes themselves normally express few MHC class I molecules, and no MHC class II molecules. It has been suggested that this limited MHC expression could play a role in the relative tolerance of liver allografts (Davies 1976, Settaf 1988). However, aberrant expression of MHC class I molecules has been observed on hepatocytes in immune-mediated diseases such as viral hepatitis and liver allograft rejection (So 1987, Steinhoff 1988). There is also some evidence that cholestasis induces hepatocyte MHC class I expression (Innes 1988). In addition, allograft rejection is also characterized by abnormal expression of MHC class II molecules on bile ducts (So 1987, Steinhoff 1988). The immunogenicity of the liver could therefore vary in these pathologic situations, and has been poorly characterized (Ferry 1987, Nossal 1989).

2. Clonal deletion.

Absence of donor-specific cytotoxic T lymphocytes (CTL) in liver-allografted recipients is suggestive of clonal deletion of these cells (Davies 1983, Houssin 1983). Such deletion could occur in the graft itself. Indeed, donor-specific CTL can be detected early in liver allograft (day 7) and are not found later (Davies 1983, Kamada 1985). Clonal deletion of autoreactive T lymphocytes is a well-established mechanism of self-tolerance. This classical clonal deletion takes place in the thymus and occurs during intra-uterine life. However, it has been shown that clonal deletion can also occur in adults (Nossal 1989). In this situation, deletion can be peripheral, and is currently assumed to be favored by the presence of high concentrations of antigen. It is therefore conceivable that the large antigenic mass of the liver favors this type of clonal deletion.

3. Suppressor cells.

Specific suppressor T cells (sTC) represent another important mechanism of self-tolerance. However, induction of suppressor cells can also occur in adult, and high concentrations of antigen is an important factor favoring this kind of tolerance (Nossal 1989). The large antigenic mass of the liver allograft could also favor the differentiation of sTC. sTC have been inconstantly found in liver allograft recipients in experimental models (Tsuchimoto 1987, Kamada 1985), but are thought to be an important tolerance mechanism in all types of transplantation in man.

4. Soluble immunosuppressive factors.

Induction of specific systemic tolerance by liver allografting is a rapid phenomenon; reversion of ongoing heart rejection by a liver allograft of the same specificity has been demonstrated (Kamada 1985). These data are suggestive of the presence of a specific circulating immunosuppressive factor produced by the liver allograft. Presence of a soluble circulating factor in the serum of liver allograft recipients has been demonstrated (Kamada 1986). The nature of this putative factor is unknown.

Anti-MHC class II antibodies or immune complexes containing these antibodies, and anti-idiotypic antibodies have been proposed; indeed, presence of both enhancing and antiidiotypic antibodies has been demonstrated in tolerant liver allograft recipients (Tsuchimoto 1987).

Several recent reports have emphasized the role of soluble MHC class I molecules as a putative candidate. Soluble MHC class I molecules can be detected in the serum of normal subjects (Kamada 1981). The presence of MHC class I molecules of donor origin has been demonstrated in liver allograft recipients, suggesting that the liver can release these molecules (Pollard 1990). The liver is probably not the exclusive source, since the presence of MHC class I molecules of the recipient type is also detectable in this case (Davies 1989). MHC class I molecules are rapidly released by the liver after hepatic transplantation (30-60 min), and are short-lived (Pollard 1990). Soluble MHC class I molecules have a smaller molecular weight than complete molecules, suggesting the deletion of the transmembranous part of the molecule. Secretion of soluble forms of MHC class I molecules could be the result of an alternative splicing of MHC class I mRNA, leading to the suppression of the transmembranous sequence of the molecule, or from a shedding of the extramembranous portion of entire molecules. Soluble MHC class I molecules are thought to favor tolerance by suppressing CTL activity or inducing specific sTC. However, conflicting data have been published on their immune effects (Priestley 1989), and more information is necessary to be sure that they play any role in liver-induced tolerance.

5. Effect of the recipient liver.

In contrast to the tolerance induced by orthotopic liver transplantation, a heterotopic auxiliary liver allograft is rapidly rejected and does not induce donor-specific tolerance (Gugenheim 1981). To explain this discrepancy, it has been suggested that immunosuppressive agents, probably released in the recipient by the liver allograft, could be removed by the recipient's own liver (Gugenheim 1981, Everson 1977). We have also shown that tolerance cannot be transferred from a liver-allografted tolerant rat 1 to a normal rat 2 using a parabiosis model; indeed, in rat 2, heart rejection occurred rapidly, while there was no histological evidence of liver rejection in the parabiosed rat 1. Furthermore, *in vitro* analyses of the reactivity to the donor haplotype confirmed the tolerant state of the liver-grafted rat 1, contrasting with the sensitized state of the heart-grafted rat 2 (Dousset, manuscript in preparation). A possible explanation for these experimental results could be the persistence of the own liver in the parabiosed animal 2, leading to the neutralization of immunosuppressive agents released by the liver allograft in rat 1. Some data suggest that Kupffer cells might play a role in the clearance of immunosuppressive substances, since inactivation of Kupffer cells by substances such as carrageenan could delay allograft rejection (Everson 1977).

REFERENCES

Iwatsuki S, Iwaki Y, Kano T, et al. Successful liver transplantation from crossmatch positive donors. Transplant Proc 1981; 13: 286.

Houssin D, Gigou M, Franco D, et al. Specific transplantation tolerance induced by spontaneously tolerated liver allograft in inbred strains of rats. Transplantation 1980; 29: 418.

Houssin D, Charpentier B, Gugenheim J, et al. Spontaneous long term acceptance of RT1 incompatible liver allografts in inbred rats. Transplantation 1983; 36: 615.

Zimmerman FA, Davies HS, Knoll PP, Gokel JM, Schmidt T. Orthotopic liver allograft in the rat. The influence of strain combination on the fate of the graft. Transplantation 1984; 37: 406.

Kamada N. Transplantation tolerance and immunosuppression following liver grafting in rats. Immunol Today 1985; 6: 336.

Nossal GJV. Immunologic tolerance. In : Fundamental immunology. Ed. Paul WE, Raven Press Ltd, New York, 1989, 571.

Hansen TH, Sachs DH. The major histocompatibility complex. In : Fundamental Immunology. Ed. PAUL WE, Raven Press Ltd, New York, 1989, 445.

Ascher NL : Effector mechanisms in allograft rejection. Transplant Proc, 1987, 19, 57.

Ferry B, Halttunen J, Leszczynski D, Schellekens H, Meide PH, Hayry P. Impact of class II major histocompatibility complex antigen expression on the immunogenic potential of isolated rat vascular endothelial cells. Transplantation, 1987, 44, 499.

Rouger P, Poupon R, Gane P, Mallissen B, Darnis F, Salmon C. Expression of blood group antigens including HLA markers in human adult liver. Tissue Antigens 1986; 27: 78.

Lautenschlager I, Taskinen E, Inkinen K, Lehto VP, Virtanen I, Hayry P. Distribution of the major histocompatibility complex antigens on different cellular components of human liver. Cell Immunol 1984; 85: 191.

Franco A, Barnaba V, Natali P, Balsano C, Musca A, Balsano F. Expression of class I and class II major histocompatibility complex antigens on human hepatocytes. Hepatology 1988; 8: 449.

Davies HSD, Taylor JE, Daniel MR, Wakerley C. Differences between pig tissues in the expression of major transplantation antigens : possible relevance for organ allografts. J Exp Med, 1976, 143, 987.

Settaf A, Milton AD, Spencer SC, Houssin D, Fabre JW. Donor class I and class II major histocompatibility complex antigen expression following liver allografting in rejecting and non rejecting rat strain combinations. Transplantation, 1988, 46, 32.

So SKS, Platt JL, Ascher NL, Snover DC. Increased expression of class I major histocompatibility complex antigen on hepatocytes in rejecting human liver allografts. Transplantation 1987; 43: 79.

Steinhoff G, Wonigeit K, Pichlmayr R. Analysis of sequential changes in major histocompatibility complex expression in human liver grafts after transplantation. Transplantation 1988; 45: 394.

Innes GK, Nagafuchi Y, Fuller BJ, Hobbs KEF. Increased expression of major histocompability antigens in the liver as a result of cholestasis. Transplantation 1988 ; 45 :749.

Davies HS, Kamada N, Roser BJ. Mechanisms of donor-specific unresponsiveness induced by liver grafting. Transplant Proc, 1983, 15, 831.

Tsuchimoto S, Kakita A, Uchino J, Mizuno K, Niiyama T, Fujii H, Matsuno Y, Natori T, Aizawa M. Mechanism of tolerance in rat liver transplantation. The role of humoral immunosuppressive factors. Transplant Proc 1987, 19, 3064.

Kamada N, Shinomiya T, Tamaki T, Ishiguro K. Immunosuppressive activity of serum from liver-grafted rats. Transplantation, 1986, 42, 581.

Tsuchimoto S, Kakita A, Uchino J, Mizuno K, Niiyama T, Fujii H, Matsuno Y, Natori T, Aizawa M. Mechanism of tolerance in rat liver transplantation. Evidence for the existence of suppressor cells. Transplant Proc 1987, 19, 514.

Pollard SG, Davies HS, Calne RY. Peroperative appearance of serum class I antigen during liver transplantation. Transplantation 1990, 49, 659.

Davies HS, Pollard SG, Calne RY. Soluble HLA antigens in the circulation of liver graft recipients. Transplantation, 1989, 47, 524.

Priestley CA, Dalchau R, Sawyer GJ, Fabre JW. A detailed analysis of the potential of water-soluble classical class I MHC molecules for the suppression of kidney allograft rejection and in vitro cytotoxic T cell responses. Transplantation 1989; 48: 1031.

Gugenheim J, Houssin D, Tamisier D, et al. Spontaneous long-term survival of liver allograft in inbred rats. Influence of the hepatectomy of the recipient's own liver. Transplantation 1981; 32: 445.

Everson NW, Stacey RL, Bell PRF. Effect of λ-carrageenan on the survival of rat heart transplants. Transplantation 1977; 24 : 393.

Immunological indices of human liver allograft rejection

David H. Adams

Liver Unit Research Laboratories, Queen Elizabeth Hospital, Edgbaston, Birmingham B152TH, UK

Address for correspondence : Selly Oak Hospital, Raddlebarn Road, Selly Oak, Birmingham, UK

Summary
Several indices of immunological activity have been studied in an attempt to find a sensitive and specific diagnostic marker for graft rejection after liver transplantation. Elevated serum levels of lymphocyte activation products such as the soluble interleukin 2 receptor are found but are non-specific. However the biliary level of SIL2R is both a sensitive and specific test for rejection which becomes elevated 24 hours before the onset of clinical features of rejection. Cytokines such as TNF, IL1 and gamma IFN have also been measured in serum but were found to be non-specific and have not been detected in bile.

Markers of graft damage also increase during rejection. B2M, part of the class 1 molecule is shed into bile during episodes of rejection and the bile/serum ratio of B2M is a sensitive and specific test for rejection. Other markers of biliary epithelial damage such as secretory component and epithelial membrane antigen can be detected in bile but are non-specific. Evidence of hepatic endothelial damage is reflected by elevated serum levels of hyaluronic acid during rejection. In addition to being a marker of acute rejection particularly high levels of HA, presumably reflecting more severe endothelial cell damage, predict a failure to respond to increased immunosuppression.

Introduction
Over the last 10 years the histological features of graft rejection after human liver transplantation have been well described allowing the differentiation of rejection from other causes of graft dysfunction on histologic grounds (Wight and Portman 1987; Hubscher et al 1985; Snover et al 1987; Ascher et al 1988). However liver biopsy cannot be carried out daily and is therefore used to confirm a clinical suspicion of rejection rather than to diagnose it *de novo*. A sensitive and specific marker of acute rejection which could be readily measured in patients on a daily basis would therefore be of great potential benefit in the management of graft dysfunction.

The rejection process can be regarded as an inflammatory cascade which starts with the presentation of transplant antigens to the host immune system leading to immune activation, the recruitment of several effector mechanisms and ultimately graft damage (Hayry 1984; Ascher 1984; Adams 1990; Sanfilippo 1988). The immunological events which accompany each step of the process can potentially be monitored as indices of immune activation and rejection.

Lymphocyte activation
The recognition of donor transplant antigens by the host immune system results in the

activation of host helper T cells. Lymphocyte activation is accompanied by functional and phenotypic changes in the cell. Activated cells express activation markers on their membrane and secrete an array of cytokines which are involved in the recruitment, activation and control of other arms of the immune response (Raulet and Bevan 1982; Wagner et al 1982; Heidecke et al 1984). Such a process might result in quantitative and qualitative changes in circulating lymphocyte subsets and several workers have attempted to determine whether such changes are specific to the rejection process (Herrod et al 1986, Herrod et al 1988; Munn et al 1988; Hathaway et al 1990). However whilst it is generally agreed that lymphocyte counts increase during rejection this is non-specific and no study has reported a pattern in lymphocyte subset composition of peripheral blood which is a reliable indicator of graft rejection.

The measurement of lymphocyte activation products would appear to offer a method of monitoring lymphocyte activation. Unfortunately two of the most important of these, the cytokines gamma interferon and interleukin 2, have proved difficult to measure in biological fluids. Tilg et al (1990) measured a number of cytokines in serum after transplantation, however whilst they found that gamma interferon, beta-2-microglobulin and neopterin were elevated they were not specific for rejection and they were unable to detect IL2. Other studies have shown a lack of specificity for serum B2M and neopterin (Maury et al 1984; Oldhafer et al 1988). In addition to secreting cytokines activated lymphocytes also release soluble forms of many of their surface antigens during activation. These include the receptor for interleukin 2 which is expressed on the cell surface in increased amounts during lymphocyte activation (Uchiyama et al 1981). The interaction of IL2 and the membrane receptor results in lymphocyte proliferation. The receptor is also shed in a stable, soluble form into the surrounding tissues and this soluble IL2 receptor (SIL2R) can be readily measured (Rubin et al 1985). Two studies have reported elevated plasma levels of SIL2R during rejection however both concluded that this elevation was not specific for rejection being also seen during infective complications in the absence of detectable rejection (Adams et al 1989a; Perkins et al 1989). Histologically the inflammatory response of rejection is centred on small bile ducts in the portal tracts and an externally draining T tube is left in place for several weeks following liver transplantation. Bile is therefore easy to sample following transplantation and offers direct access to the site of the rejection process. There is evidence that the analysis of bile provides a more accurate reflection of the immune events of rejection than does the analysis of serum since biliary levels of SIL2R were far more sensitive and specific markers of rejection than the corresponding serum levels (Adams et al 1989a).

Lymphocyte recruitment
Lymphocytes probably accumulate at the site of rejection by a combination of proliferation in situ and recruitment from the periphery in response to locally secreted chemotactic factors (Ascher et al 1983 and 1984; Kupiec-Weglinski et al 1985; Adams 1990). Such factors have been demonstrated in bile after liver transplantation (Adams et al 1989b) and specific lymphocyte chemotactic factors appear to be secreted early in the rejection process (Hathaway et al 1990). Further studies have demonstrated that these factors show preferential activity for host CD8 T cells and are probably secreted by CD4 helper T cells (Hathaway et al 1991). In addition host lymphocytes show increased chemotactic activity *in vitro* to standard chemotactic factors prior to episodes of clinical rejection. The studies published to date have been concerned with the mechanisms of rejection rather than in the use of *in vitro* chemotactic assays as a diagnostic tool. However, a simplified *in vitro* chemotaxis assay using 48 well microchemotaxis chambers can produce a semiquantitative result within 6 hours (Richards and McCullough 1984) and therefore has potential as a monitor of immune activation.

Effector mechanisms
Liver damage in graft rejection is probably mediated by several different effector mechanisms. These include cytotoxic T cells, antibody secretion and the activation of other immune cells such as eosinophils, neutrophils and monocytes (Sanfillipo 1988; Adams 1990).

Donor specific lymphocyte-mediated cytotoxicity to donor spleen cells can be detected in vitro after transplantation although the development of such responses is not specific enough to be used to diagnose clinical rejection (Grant et al 1986). Activated cytotoxic T cells with specificity for donor HLA antigens can be isolated from liver biopsies during rejection (Fung et al 1986; Markus et al 1988) and CD8 positive cells are found infiltrating target structures such as bile ducts in liver biopsies (McCaughan et al 1990). The isolation of T cell clones from liver biopsies takes several days and cannot therefore be used for daily monitoring of immunological activity. However, activated CD8 positive T cells shed a soluble form of the CD8 receptor which can be measured in biological fluids. Early results from our Unit suggest that plasma levels of soluble CD8 rise before episodes of rejection whereas no rise is seen in patients who fail to develop rejection (Hathaway and Adams unpublished observations). Whether soluble CD8 is also elevated in viral and bacterial infections after transplantation is yet to be determined but seems likely.

Studies demonstrating increased levels of circulating donor specific antibodies provide evidence for the involvement of humoral mechanisms (Donaldson et al 1987; Bryan et al 1988). During episodes of acute rejection local secretion into bile of immunoglobulins (particularly IgM and IgG) occurs although the low specificity and sensitivity of such findings precludes their use as diagnostic tests (Adams et al 1990a). Monitoring the development of donor specific antibodies after transplantation might provide a useful diagnostic test in the future.

Peripheral blood neutrophils become activated during episodes of acute rejection when they show increased chemotactic responses and an enhanced secretion of superoxide radicals and proteolytic enzymes *in vitro*. Similar activation was not seen in patients who failed to reject their grafts (Adams et al 1990b). These findings are in keeping with the histological observations that large numbers of neutrophils are present within the portal infiltrate during rejection (Wight and Portman 1987; Hubscher et al 1985). However, it is likely that neutrophils will also be activated during infective episodes, particularly bacterial cholangitis reducing the diagnostic specificity of neutrophil function tests.

Large numbers of eosinophils are seen in the portal tract inflammatory infiltrate during rejection episodes and Sankary et al (1989) used multivariate analysis to demonstrate that their presence was a strong histological indicator of rejection. In addition the same group have shown that peripheral blood eosinophil counts rise prior to episodes of rejection and that this rise is both sensitive and specific for rejection (Foster et al 1989). Thus a simple differential white cell count might be a powerful diagnostic tool to differentiate rejection from other causes of graft dysfunction.

Monocytes and macrophages are also present in the inflammatory infiltrate of rejection (Wight and Portman 1987; Hubscher et al 1985, Hofman et al 1991). Activated macrophages secrete many cytokines one of which is tumour necrosis factor alpha and three studies have reported elevated serum levels of TNFa during rejection episodes (Adams et al 1990; Imagawa et al 1990; Tilg et al 1990). However the specificity of elevated TNF levels for rejection is poor reflecting the release of this cytokine in response to a wide variety of stimulants.

Target damage
The important targets for the inflammatory response in acute rejection are the biliary epithelium, venous endothelium and much less importantly hepatocytes (Wight and Portman 1987; Hubscher et al 1985; Snover et al 1987). In chronic or ductopenic rejection arterial endothelium is invariably involved in the characteristic arteriopathy (Portman et al 1983; Vierling et al 1985).

Evidence for bile duct damage can be found by measuring markers of biliary epithelial damage. Two proteins which are confined to the biliary epithelium in the liver are epithelial membrane antigen and secretory component. EMA can be detected in bile after liver transplantation but the levels do not rise with rejection. Free secretory component is shed into bile during rejection when increased amounts can be detected but is also increased during infective complications such as bacterial cholangitis reducing its specificity as a diagnostic tool (Adams et al 1987). Lymphocyte mediated bile duct damage is probably directed at HLA class 1 molecules which are expressed strongly on bile ducts after transplantation (Steinhoff 1990; Hubscher et al 1989). Class I molecules are expressed on the cell surface in association with beta 2 micro- globulin (Bach and Van Rood 1976). Serum levels of beta-2-microglobulin are non-specifically elevated during rejection which probably reflects its release from lymphocytes and the effect of renal function on B2M clearance (Maury et al 1984; Adams et al 1988; Tilg et al 1990). However in one study biliary levels were found to be far more specific for rejection (Adams et al 1988). Other studies have demonstrated release of soluble class I antigens into serum during rejection and into bile after transplantation although the numbers of patients studied were too small to assess the sensitivity and specificity (Pollard et al 1989).

Evidence of hepatic endothelial cell damage has been sought by measuring serum levels of hyaluronic acid, a proteoglycan which is removed from the circulation by hepatic endothelial cells. Circulating levels are elevated 24 hours before clinical episodes of rejection and tend to be higher during rejection than during other complications (Adams et al 1989c).

Assessment of prognosis using immunological indices.
Whilst most rejection episodes respond satisfactorily to treatment with high-dose corticosteroids 5-10% of patients will develop irreversible rejection (Ascher et al 1988; Pichlmayr & Gubernatis 1987; Adams & Neuberger 1990). At present it is not possible to predict which patients will progress. The histological features and the composition of the inflammatory infiltrate may give some clues (Snover et al 1987; Perkins et al 1988). A serological test which predicted response to treatment would be useful since it would allow one to select those patients with irreversible rejection at a stage when they might be potentially more responsive to treatment. Very high levels of the bile duct derived enzyme gamma glutamyl transferase have been associated with the development of irreversible rejection (Lasky et al 1984) as have high levels of hyaluronic acid (presumably reflecting endothelial damage) (Adams et al 1990) and tumour necrosis factor alpha (presumably an indicator of immune activation) (Adams et al 1990).

References

Adams DH, Burnett D, Stockley RA, P McMaster and Elias E (1987). Markers of biliary epithelial damage in liver allograft rejection. Transplant. Proc. 19: 3820-3821.
Adams DH, Burnett D, Hubscher SG, Stockley R, McMaster P, Elias E (1988). Biliary beta-2-microglobulin in liver allograft rejection. Hepatology; 8: 1565-1570.
Adams DH, Wang L, Hubscher SG, Elias E, Neuberger JM (1989a). Soluble interleukin-2 receptors in serum and bile of liver transplant recipients. Lancet; i: 469-472.
Adams DH, Burnett D, Stockley RA, Elias E (1989b). Patterns of leucocyte chemotaxis after liver transplantation. Gastroenterology; 97:   433-438.
Adams DH, Wang L, Hubscher SG, Neuberger JM (1989c). Hepatic endothelial cells: targets in liver allograft rejection? Transplantation 1989; 47: 479-482.
Adams DH (1990). Mechanisms of human liver allograft rejection. Clin Sci. 78: 343-350.
Adams DH, Neuberger JM (1990). Patterns of liver allograft rejection. J. Hepatol. 10: 113-119.
Adams DH, Hubscher SG, Burnett D, Elias E (1990a). Immunoglobulins in liver allograft rejection: evidence for deposition and secretion within the liver. Transplant. Proc. 22: 1834-1835.
Adams DH, Wang LF, Burnett D, Stockley RA, Neuberger JM (1990b). Neutrophil activation: an important cause of tissue damage during liver allograft rejection? Transplantation; 50: 86-91.

Adams DH, Garner C, Neuberger JM (1990c). Serum tumour necrosis factor alpha in liver transplantation. Transplant Proc; 22: 2310.

Ascher NL, Chen S, Hoffman RA, et al (1983). Maturaration of cytotoxic T cells within sponge matrix allografts. J. Immunol. 131: 617-621.

Ascher NL, Hoffman RA, Hanto DW, Simmons RL (1984). Cellular basis of allograft rejection. Immunol. Rev. 77: 217-232.

Ascher NL, Stock PG, Bumgardner GI, Payne WD and Najarian JS (1988). Infection and rejection of primary hepatic transplants in 93 consecutive patients. Surg. Gynecol. Obstet. 167: 474-484.

Ascher NL, Freese DK, Paradis K, Snover DC, Bloomer JR (1988). Rejection of the transplanted liver. In: Maddrey WC ed. Transplantation of the Liver. New York; Elsevier; 167-189.

Bach FH and Van Rood JJ (1976). The major histocompatibility complex - genetics and biology. N. Eng. J. Med. 295; 806-813.

Bryan CF, Newman JT, Tilquist RL, Husberg B, Klintmalm GB, Stone MJ (1987). Development of class I-directed lymphocytotoxic antibodies after liver transplantation. Transplant. Proc. 19: 2392-2393.

Donaldson PT, Alexander GJM, O'Grady J et al (1987). Evidence of an immune response to HLA class 1 antigens in the vanishing bile duct syndrome after liver transplantation. Lancet; i: 945-948.

Foster P, Sankary S, Hart M, Ashmann M, Williams JW (1989). Blood and graft eosinophilia as predictors of rejection in human liver transplantation. Transplantation; 47: 72-74.

Fung JJ, Zeevi A, Starzl TE, Iwatsuki S, Duquesnoy RJ (1986). Functional characterization of infiltrating T lymphocytes in human hepatic allografts. Hum. Immunol. 16: 182-199.

Grant D, Wall W, Stiller C, Keown P, Duff J, Ghent C (1986). Immunologic monitoring for rejection after liver transplantation. Transplant. Proc. 18: 171-173.

Hathaway M, Adams DH, Burnett D, Elias E (1990). Recruitment of lymphocytes to human liver allografts during rejection. Transplant. Proc. 22: 2306-2307.

Hathaway M, Adams DH, Burnett D, Elias E (1991). Secretion into bile of chemotactic factors for CD8+ lymphocytes during rejection of human liver allografts. Transplant. Proc. 23: 1424-1425.

Hayry P, von Willebrand E, Parthenais E, Nemlander A, Soots A, Lautenschlager I, Alfoldy P, Renkonen R (1984). The inflammatory mechanisms of allograft rejection. Immunol. Rev. 77: 85-142.

Heidecke CD, Kupiec-Weglinski JW, Lear DA et al (1984). Interactions between T lymphocyte subsets supported by IL2 rich lymphokines produce acute rejection of vascularised cardiac allografts in T cell deprived rats. J. Immunol. 133: 582-588.

Herrod HG, Williams JW, Valenski WR, Vera S (1986). Serial Immunologic studies in recipients of hepatic allografts. Clin. Immunol. Immunopath. 40: 298-304.

Herrod HG, Williams JW, Dean PJ (1988). Alterations in immunologic measurements in patients experiencing early hepatic allograft rejection. Transplantation; 45: 923-925.

Hoffman M, Wonigeit K, Behrend M, et al. Tissue distribution of IL1 beta and TNF alpha producing cells in rejecting liver allografts. Transplant. Proc. 23: 1421-1423.

Hubscher SG, Clements D, Elias E, McMaster P (1985). Biopsy findings in cases of rejection of liver allografts. J. Clin. Pathol. 38: 1366-1373.

Hubscher SG, Adams DH, Elias E (1988). Beta-2-microglobulin expression in the liver after liver transplantation. J. Clin. Pathol. 41: 1049-1057.

Hubscher SG (1991). Histological findings in liver allograft rejection - new insights into the pathogenesis of hepatocellular damage in liver allografts. Histopathol (in press).

Imagawa DK, Millis JM, Olthoff KM et al (1990). The role of tumour necrosis factor in allograft rejection. 1 Evidence that elevated levels of tumour necrosis factor alpha predict rejection following liver transplantation. Transplantation; 50: 219-225.

Kupiec-Weglinski JW, de Sousa M, Tilney NL (1985). The importance of lymphocyte migration patterns in experimental organ transplantation. Transplantation; 40: 1-6.

Lasky S, Demetris AJ, Dekker A, et al (1984). Glutamyl transpeptidase as a marker for rejection following liver transplantation. Hepatology; 4: 1045-1047.

Ludwig J, Weisner RH, Batts KP, Perkins JP, RAF Krom (1987). The acute vanishing bile duct syndrome (acute irreversible rejection) after orthotopic liver transplantation. Hepatology; 7: 476-483.

Markus BH, Demetris AJ, Saidman S, Fung JJ, Zeevi A, Starzl TE, Duquesnoy RJ (1988). Alloreactive T lymphocytes cultured from liver transplant biopsies: Associations of HLA specificity with clinicopathological findings. Clin. Transplant. 2: 70-75.

Maury CPJ, Hockerstedt K, Tepo A-M, Lautenschlager I, Scheinin TM (1984). Changes in serum amyloid A protein and beta-2-microglobulin in association with liver allograft rejection. Transplantation; 38: 551-553.

McCaughan GW, Davies JS, Wuagh JA, Bishop GA et al. A quantitative analysis of T lymphocyte populations in human liver allografts undergoing rejection: the use of monoclonal antibodies and double immunolabeling. Hepatology 1990; 12: 1305-1313.

Munn SR, Tominaga S, Perkins JD, Hayes DH, Weisner RH, Krom RAK (1988). Increasing peripheral T lymphocyte counts predict rejection in human liver allografts. Transplant. Proc. 20 (suppl 1): 674-675.

Oldhafer KJ, Schaefer O, Wonigict K, Ringe B, Pichlmayr R (1988). Monitoring of serum neopterin levels after liver transplantation. Transplant. Proc. 20: 671-673.

Perkins JD, Rakela J, Sterioff S, Banks PM, Weisner RH, Krom RAF (1988). Results of treatment in hepatic allograft rejection depend on the immunohistologic pattern of the portal T lymphocyte infiltrate. Transplant. Proc. 20: 223-225.

Perkins JD, Nelson DL, Rakela J, Grambasch PM, Krom RAF (1989). Soluble interleukin-2 receptor level as an indicator of liver allograft rejection. Transplantation 1989; 47:77-81.

Pichlmayr R, Gubernatis G (1987). Rejection of the liver and review of current immunosuppressive protocols. Transplantation Proc; 19: 4367-4369.

Pollard SG, Davies H FFS, Calne RY (1989). Soluble class I antigen in human bile. Transplantation 1989; 48: 712-714.

Portman B, Neuberger JM, Williams R (1983). Intrahepatic bile duct lesions. In Liver Transplantation: The Cambridge/King's College Hospital experience. Calne RY ed New York: Grune and Stratton; 279-287.

Raulet DH, Bevan MJ (1982). A differentiation factor required for the expression of cytotoxic T cell function. Nature 1982; 296: 754-757.

Richards KL, McCullough J (1984). A Modified microchemotaxis chamber method for chemotaxis and chemokinesis. Immunol. Comm. 1984, 13; 49-62.

Rubin LA, Kurman CC, Fritz ME et al (1985). Soluble interleukin-2 receptors are released from activated human lymphoid cells *in vitro*. J. Immunology 135: 3172-7.

Sanfilippo F (1988). Immunology of liver transplantation. In W.C. Maddrey ed: Transplantation of liver. Elsevier (Amsterdam); 219-248.

Sankary S, Foster P, Hart M et al (1989). An analysis of the determinants of hepatic allograft rejection using step-wise logistic regression. Transplantation; 47: 74-77.

Snover DC, Freese D, Sharp HL, Bloomer JR, Najarian JS, Ascher NL (1987). Liver allograft rejection. An analysis of the use of biopsy in determining the outcome of rejection. Am. J. Surg. Pathol. 11: 1-10.

Steinhoff G. Major histocompatibility antigens in human liver transplants. J. Hepatol. 1990; 11: 9-15.

Tilg H, Vogel W, Aulitsky WE et al (1990). Evaluation of cytokines and cytokine-induced secondary messages in sera of patients after liver transplantation. Transplantation; 49: 1074-1080.

Uchiyama T, Broder S, Waldmann TA (1981). A monoclonal antibody (anti-TAC) reactive with activated and functionally mature human T cells. J. Immunol. 126: 1393-1397.

Vierling JM, Fennell RH (1985). Histopathology of early and late human hepatic allograft rejection: evidence of destruction of interlobular bile ducts. Hepatology 1985; 5: 1076-1082

Wagner H, Hardt C, Riouse BT, Rollinghoff M, Scheurich P, Pfizenmeir K (1982). Dissection of the proliferative and differentiative signals controlling murine cytotoxic T lymphocyte responses. J. Exp. Med. 155: 1876-1881.

Wight DGD, Portman B (1987). Pathology of liver transplantation. In Liver transplantation. Calne RY ed. London: Grune & Stratton: 385-412.

Immunological, metabolic and infectious aspects of liver transplantation. Eds D.A. Vuitton, C. Balabaud, D. Houssin, D. Dhumeaux. John Libbey Eurotext, Paris © 1991, pp. 49-57.

Cytological techniques in the follow-up of liver transplants

Krister Höckerstedt, Irmeli Lautenschlager[1]

IV Department of Surgery and its Transplantation Laboratory [1], University of Helsinki, Kasarmikatu 11, 00130 Helsinki, Finland

Acute rejection is seen in some 70% of liver grafts (1). Early diagnosis is important because the rejection may destroy the transplant. Identification of the immunological process is difficult since the clinical signs and symptoms are very unspecific. Usually impairment of liver function is seen, which can mimick anything from rejection to cholestasis, cholangitis or other infections — both bacterial, viral and fungal. It is not possible to establish a correct diagnosis without a biopsy sample from the graft. Two methods are available. A core biopsy reveals the histology and fine needle aspiration method of Helsinki (FNAB) gives you the cytological picture of the immunological events in the graft. The morphological picture varies in acute rejection which has been well described by Wight and Portman (2). But, such a core biopsy carries a risk of bleeding complications, particularly in the patients with decreased liver function and a severely impaired clotting profile. Liver hematoma, sepsis, lung empyema and even death of the patient have been reported in connection with histological liver biopsies (1,3). We describe the experience with FNAB in liver transplant patients in Helsinki.

Technical performance of FNAB.

The FNAB is an atraumatic procedure, which can be repeated daily if wanted. The technique was primarily developed for identification of acute rejection in kidney transplant patients in Helsinki (4–6) and more than 12.000 renal specimens have already been studied. The method is now used in some 50 transplant centers. The technique in liver transplantation is similar to the one for kidney transplants. The skin is penetrated from the medial part of the right costal margin and the liver is punctured. Ultrasound (US) guidance is adviceable only if the patient has major ascites and the liver is small, otherwise not. We have used US guidance in < 2 % of the cases. The technique is described in detail in Table 1.

Table 1. Technique of FNAB in Liver Transplant Patients

1. Use a 0.5 mm OD spinal needle (25-gauge 3½ inch)
2. Puncture the skin of the abdomen just below the medial part of the right costal margin. No local anesthesia or radiology guidance is needed
3. Direct needle 30° upward and 30° to the right
4. Instruct patient to take a normal breath and hold it
5. Insert the needle into the liver
6. Remove mandrin and attach a syringe containing culture medium to the needle
7. Aspirate a specimen while slowly moving the needle to and fro in short 1 cm movements inside the liver
8. Release the negative pressure in syringe
9. Instruct patient to breathe
10. Rinse the aspirated sample twice in injection needle holder (cuvette) and aspirate the whole sample into syringe and close its tip
11. Transfer a blood drop from tip of finger into a smaller syringe as control

The cytocentrifuge preparations of the two 10–20 μl specimens are stained with May–Grünwald–Giemsa (MGG), and quantitation of inflammation is done using an increment method (6, 7). The idea is to detect the inflammatory cells invading the graft during rejection, cells which are not equally abundant in the blood. The intensity of inflammation can be numerically graded to form a "total corrected increment" (TCI), which is the sum of corrected increment values of the aspirate after subtracting the blood background. The inflammatory cells with the highest diagnostic value of acute rejection, i.e. lymphoid blasts, plasma cells, monoblasts and macrophages have a correcting factor of 1.0, whereas those of less importance are labelled with a factor of 0.1 or 0.2. The specimen are considered representative if they contain >7 hepatocytes per 100 leukocytes counted. The condition of the hepatocytes is evaluated and graded from 1 to 4; 1 is normal and 4 means necrosis. Observation of bile droplets or vacualization of the cells is reported. The results are ready in 2 hours. We would like to stress that we use the

FNAB method in the daily clinical work affecting immediately the treatment of patients.

The first FNAB is obtained at surgery and hence every 1-3 days during the hospital period after transplantation. After the first month the biopsies are taken only when deterioration of liver function or unexplained fever is seen. It should be noted that the FNAB method is of no value in the estimation of chronic rejection, where a morphological diagnosis from a core biopsy is mandatory.

Since our first experimental (8) and clinical (9) experience in 1984 more than 1500 FNAB specimens have been obtained from 87 liver grafts in Helsinki. 87% of these aspiration biopsies were successful (10). The main reasons for failure were a sample containing too much blood, too few hepatocytes, or intraperitoneal conta-mination. In case a sample is inadequate a new one may be obtained the same day. Absolutely no complications have been seen, not even pain. The lack of complications has also been reported by the Innsbruck group, who was the first to adopt our technique (11), and others (12).

Diagnosis of acute rejection

Basic immunosuppression in our center has been triple drug therapy; methylprednisolone (MP), azathioprine (Aza) and Cyclosporine A (CyA). In four patients OKT-3 prophylaxis was given for the first 13 days instead of CyA. It should be noted that neither graft preservation nor the transplant surgery in itself does to any greater extent affect the immune response seen in FNAB. In the early postoperative phase the TCI score is usually < 2.0. Thus, a TCI score >3 including lymphoid blast cells and lymphocytosis in the liver specimen is considered as onset of immunological activation of acute rejection. If the rejection is severe and continues, the cellular infiltrate becomes dominated by mononuclear phagocytes. Appearance of large numbers of macrophages is usually associated with irreversible rejection (13, 14). It should be stressed that the cellular picture of a blood specimen is totally different and practically no blast cells or activated lymphocytes are found during rejection (7). FNAB provides signs of acute rejection 1-4 days before elevation of s-bilirubin, s-alkaline phosphatase or s-ALAT is seen (15) We have also found synchronous elevation of the serum acute phase proteins orosomucoids and a-1-antichymotrypsin, but not of C-reactive protein (CRP), in connection with acute rejection (16).

We believe that the diagnosis of acute rejection is appropriate only when clinical signs of liver dysfunction occur concomitantly. Thus, in unclear cases the cytological graft specimen should be repeated the same or the following day.

```
HUCS, IV Department of Surgery. Transplantation laboratory
Patient: n.n.
Biopsy no: 1519          day: June 5, 1991    Days after tx: 7

+---------------------------------+------+-------+------+------+
I Solut = cells                   I Fnab I Blood I Cf   I Co.i I
+---------------------------------+------+-------+------+------+
I LYMFOBLASTIT                    I 0    I 0     I 1    I 0    I
+---------------------------------+------+-------+------+------+
I PLASMABLASTIT JA PLASMASOLUI 3  I 0    I 1     I 3    I
+---------------------------------+------+-------+------+------+
I AKT.LYMFOSYYTIT                 I 4    I 0     I .5   I 2    I
+---------------------------------+------+-------+------+------+
I LGL LYMFOSYYTIT                 I 1    I 1     I .2   I 0    I
+---------------------------------+------+-------+------+------+
I PIENET LYMFOSYYTIT              I 30   I 13    I .1   I 1.7  I
+---------------------------------+------+-------+------+------+
I PMN JUV                         I 0    I 0     I .1   I 0    I
+---------------------------------+------+-------+------+------+
I PMN NEUTRO                      I 47   I 60    I .1   I 0    I
+---------------------------------+------+-------+------+------+
I PMN BASO                        I 0    I 2     I .1   I 0    I
+---------------------------------+------+-------+------+------+
I PMN EOS                         I 7    I 14    I .1   I 0    I
+---------------------------------+------+-------+------+------+
I MONOBLASTIT                     I 0    I 0     I 1    I 0    I
+---------------------------------+------+-------+------+------+
I MONOSYYTIT                      I 8    I 10    I .2   I 0    I
+---------------------------------+------+-------+------+------+
I MAKROFAAGIT                     I 0    I       I 1    I 0    I
+---------------------------------+------+-------+------+------+
I TCI                                                   I 6.7  I
+--------------------------------------------------------+-----+

Tissue cells                    20   Morphology 1.      1
Bile in hepatocytes              1   Morphology 2.      2
Cya deposits in hepatocytes          Morph. mean        1.5
------------------------------------------------------------
Lausunto:
MAKSASIIRRÄNNÄISEN ONB-NÄYTE ON EDUSTAVA, SIINÄ NÄHDÄÄN RUNSAASTI PAREN-
KYYMISOLUJA.    HEPATOSYYTEISSÄ EI JUURI PALJOAKAAN MORFOLOGISIA MUUTOKSIA
NÄHDÄ, SAPPEA SEN SIJAAN HAVAITAAN PIENIÄ MÄÄRIÄ.
LYMFOSYYTTEJÄ ON ONB-NÄYTTEESSÄ RUNSAASTI, SELVÄSTI YLI VEREN TASON,
JOUKOSSA AKTIVOITUNEITA MUOTOJA JA LUKUISIA BLASTEJA (N. 20 BLASTIA/
PREP.).    MONOSYYTTISARJAN SOLUJA ON NÄYTTEESSÄ VEREN TASOA VASTATEN.
*
YHTEENVETO:
VERESSÄ LYMFOPENIA, EI BLASTEJA.    VERESSÄ HUOMATTAVA EOSINOFILIA.
SELVÄ IMMUNOAKTIVAATIO GRAFTISSA.    LYMFOSYTOOSI JA BLASTIRESPONSSI
SEKÄ VEREN EOSINOFILIA SOPIVAT TYYPILLISESTI AKUUTTIIN SELLULAARISEEN
REJEKTIOON.    PARENKYYMISOLUT OVAT HYVÄKUNTOISIA, MUTTA VÄHÄN SAPPEA
NÄHDÄÄN.
*
050691      IRMELI LAUTENSCHLAGER
            IL/PM.
```

Fig. 1.   A typical FNAB finding in a liver transplant patient revealing acute rejection. The FNAB of the graft contains plasma blastas and plasma cells and the *Total Corrected Increment* (TCI) is 6.7 .

In patients with ascites contamination is possible so that intraperitoneal cells and often also mesothelial cells may be aspirated into the specimen distubing the interpretention of the FNAB. These cells must be identified and a new sample obtained, where no suction in the syringe should be maintained when the needle is withdrawn from the liver.

Acute rejection was noted in 68% of the transplants. In all but two grafts the rejection occurred within 21 days post-transplant (mean 9 days, range 4 to 27 days). Fig. 1 shows the FNAB report from our transplant laboratory of a patient with acute rejection. Two periods of rejection were noted in four patients, 7 – 32 days after the first one. In three patients even three acute rejection periods have occurred. In Fig. 1 typical inflammatory profiles are summarized from 22 reversible rejections.

Monitoring acute rejection.

The rejections have been treated with MP 3 mg/kg for five days with or without increased doses of CyA. With this antirejection treatment an acute rejection episode is usually discontinued at the stage of lymphoid response and the disappearance of the blast cells is normally seen < 3 days. Although it might be possible to stop antirejection treatment, we have continued with the regimen for a full 5 five day period. Nevertheless, at the end of the antirejection treatment period the FNAB findings should be clear on the point that the lymphoid response is vanishing. If the immune activation in the transplant continues in spite of a 5 day anti-rejection treatment, we believe that such an event needs further therapy. Our findings have been seconded by the Hannover group who particularly found the monitoring the duration of a rejection period useful making stopping of rejection treatment possible when the immunological event has subsided, and detection of steroid resistent rejection (17).

The liver tissue changes caused by rejection have usually been reflected as damage of hepatocytes in the FNAB specimens. Vacuolization and bile droplets in the hepatocytes are common findings (7). In most rejection episodes intrahepatic cholestasis is observed, too. However, cholestasis in itself is not indicative of acute rejection, as also ischemia, graft perfusion damage and other conditions may predispose to intrahepatic cholestasis (7, 18).

All but one acute rejection period have been reversible. In that particular patient the TCI peaked to a record of 50.4, and contained all the elements of a severe rejection described above. The patient was successfully retransplantated two weeks later. – Overall actuarial 1-year survival is 78%, and in our largest single patient group – PBC with 30 patients – it is 87%.

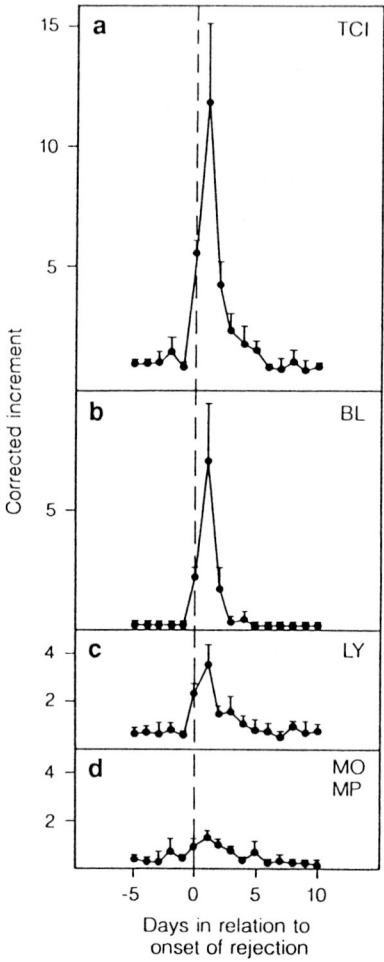

Fig. 2. **a** Inflammatory profiles of 22 episodes of rejection expressed in *corrected increment units*. **b–d** The major inflammatory cell components: **b** lymphoid blasts, **c** lymphocytes, **d** monocytes and macrophages. The onset of inflammation (day 0) is the first day with >3.0 TCI units and blast cells in the aspirate. (With kind permission from the Springer Verlag, Transplant Int 1991, 4: 54–61.)

Correlation between FNAB and histology

A close correlation of FNAB results to histology findings has been observed both in experimental (8, 14) and clinical (12, 19)) liver transplant studies. We first showed in non-immunosuppressed experimental animals that irreversible rejection occurred in one third of the pigs. The inflammatory response peaked earlier, and was more pronounced compared to changes in animals on CyA prophylaxis. The histological picture in these two groups were typical and correlated very well with these FNAB findings.

In a patient study the Birmingham group found a positive predictive value of FNAB to be 86.3 % (12). The largest liver transplant center in Paris reported an agreement between results of FNAB and histology in 16 out of 18 cases (20). In this context it is important to remind us all, that there is no 100% agreement between different pathologists on the diagnosis of acute rejection (21).

FNAB and infections

Bacterial infections do not affect the inflammatory profile of the FNAB itself, and the TCI rarely exceeds 3.0. (22). The FNAB method may also be useful in infection diagnosis as bacterial infections located in the graft may be revealed by the presence of these very same bacteria together with a large numbers of granulocytes (23).

Differentiation of acute rejection from CMV-infection may be greatly enlighted by the FNAB investigations (22, 23). CMV-disease may affect the result of FNAB by causing mild inflammation of the transplant. We found a TCI value of 3.2 ± 0.9 in a group of 7 patients with CMV disease, compared to a TCI of 12.0 ± 3.3 in 21 patients with acute rejection (23). Also, fewer blast cells and activated lymphocytes appeared in these FNAB specimens than found in acute rejection. Furthermore, the blood of the CMV-patients displayed blast cells and activated lymphocytes, not found in the blood of patients with acute rejection. The usefullness of FNAB in differentiating CMV-infection from rejection has been confirmed by the Hannover group (24). In this context it is important to remember that the diagnosis of viral infections should always be confirmed by specific virological methods.

The value of the FNAB method has recently been reviewed (25). We would like to conclude that this aspiration cytology method is not merely a research tool, we use it in the daily work with patients and its results immediately affects the treatment of the patients.

1. Ascher NL, Stock PG, Bumgardner GL et al. Infection and rejection of primary hepatic transplant in 93 consecutive patients treated with triple immunosuppressive therapy. Surg Gynecol & Obstet 1988, 167: 474–484.

2. Wight DGD, Portman B. Pathology of rejection. In: Liver transplantation. Ed. Calne RY. Grune & Stratton, London, 1987, pp 385–410.

3. Saliba F, Gugenheim J, Samuel D et al. Orthotopic liver transplantation in humans; monitoring by serial graft biopsies. Transplant Proc 1987, 19: 2454–2456.

4. Pasternack A, Virolainen M, Häyry P. Fine-needle aspiration biopsy in the diagnosis of human renal allograft rejection. J Urol 1973, 109: 167–172.

5. Willebrand E von. Fine aspiration cytology of human renal transplants. Cell Immunol Immunopathol 1980. 17: 309–320.

6. Häyry P, v Willebrand E. Practical guidelines for fine needle aspiration biopsy of human renal transplants. Ann Clin Res 1981, 13: 288–306.

7. Lautenschlager I, Höckerstedt K, Ahonen J et al. Fine-needle aspiration biopsy in the monitoring of liver allografts. II. Application to human allografts. Transplantation 1988, 46: 47–52.

8. Höckerstedt K, Lautenschlager I, Ahonen J et al. Fine needle aspiration cytology aand histology of liver allografts in the pig. In: Orthotopic liver transplantation. Ed. Krom R, Gips C. M Nijhoff Publ. The Hague, The Netherlands. 1984, pp 50–57.

9. Lautenschlager I, Höckerstedt H, Willebrand E von et al. Aspiration cytology of a human liver allograft. Transplant Proc 1984, 16: 1243–1246.

10. Höckerstedt K, Lautenschlager I. Fine needle aspiration biopsy in liver transplants. Transplant Proc 1989, 21: 3625–3626.

11. Vogel W, Margreiter R, Schmalz F et al. Preliminary results with fine needle aspiration biopsy in liver grafts. Transplant Proc 1984, 16: 1240–1242.

12. Kirby RM, Young JA, Hubscher SG et al. The accuracy of aspiration cytology in the diagnosis of rejection after orthotopic liver transplantation. Transplant Int 1988, 1: 119–126.

13. Lautenschlager I, Höckerstedt K, Taskinen E. Fine needle aspiration cytology of liver and allograft in pig. Transplantation 1984, 38: 330–334.

14. Lautenschlager I, Höckerstedt K, Taskinen E et al. Fine-needle aspiration biopsy in the monitoring of liver allografts. I. Correlation between aspiration biopsy and core biopsy in experimental pig liver allografts. Transplantation 1988, 46: 41-46.

15. Höckerstedt K, Lautenschlager I, Ahonen J et al. Diagnosis of rejection in liver transplantation. J Hepatol 1988, 6: 217-221.

16. Maury CPJ, Teppo A-M, Höckerstedt K. Acute phase proteins and liver allograft rejection. Liver 1988, 8: 75-79.

17. Nashan B, Schlitt HJ, Ringe B et al. Transplantation aspiration cytology in the diagnosis of steroid resistant rejection in liver allograft patients. Transplant Proc 1990, 22: 2297-2298.

18. Williams JW, Vera SV. Peters TG et al. Cholestatic jaundice after liver transplantation. A non-immunologically mediated event. Am J Surg 1986, 151: 165-170.

19. Greene CL, Fehrman I, Tillery GW et al. Liver transplant aspiration cytology is a useful tool for indentifying and monitoring acute rejection. Transplant Proc 1988, 20: 659-660.

20. Carbonnel F, Samuel D, Reynes M et al. Fine-needle aspiration biopsy of human liver allografts. Correlation with liver histology for the diagnosis of acute rejection. Transplantation 1990, 50: 704-707.

21. Snover DC, Freese DK, Sharp HL et al. Liver allograft rejection. An analysis of the use of biopsy in determining outcome of rejection. Am J Surg Pathol 1987, 11: 1-10.

22. Höckerstedt K, Lautenschlager I, Ahonen J et al. Differentiation between acute rejection and infection in liver transplant patients. Transplant Proc 1989, 21: 2317-2318.

23. Lautenschlager I, Höckerstedt K, Salmela K et al.Fine-needle aspiration biopsy in the monitoring of liver allografts. Different cellular findings during rejection and CMV infection. Transplantation 1990, 50: 798-803.

24. Schlitt HJ, Nashan B, Ringe Burkhard et al. Differentiation of liver graft dysfunction by transplant aspiration cytology. Transplantation 1991, 51: 786-792.

25. Lautenschlager I, Höckerstedt K, Häyry P. Fine-needle aspiration biopsy monitoring of liver allografts. Transplant Int 1991, 4: 54-61.

Immunological, metabolic and infectious aspects of liver transplantation. Eds D.A. Vuitton, C. Balabaud, D. Houssin, D. Dhumeaux. John Libbey Eurotext, Paris © 1991, pp. 59-64.

Serum secretory component and plasma hyaluronic acid levels: complementary markers of graft rejection after liver transplantation ?

C. Vanlemmens[1]*, E. Seilles[1], D.A. Vuitton[1], B. Kantelip[2], S. Bresson-Hadni[1], J. Magnette[3], G. Mantion[1], M. Gillet[1], J.P. Miguet[1]

[1] *Groupe de Recherche en Transplantation Hépatique et Immunologie Clinique, CHU Jean Minjoz, 25030 Besançon, France.* [2] *Laboratoire d'Anatomie Pathologique, CHU Jean Minjoz, 25030 Besançon, France.* [3] *Laboratoire de Pharmacologie Clinique, CHU Jean Minjoz, 25030 Besançon, France*

* *Author for correspondence*

SUMMARY

As bile duct cells and endothelial cells are the main targets in graft rejection, serum immunoreactive free secretory component (Ir F-SC) levels and plasma concentrations of hyaluronic acid (HA) were assessed simultaneously in 15 patients within the 30 days following liver transplantation. In patients with acute graft rejection, plasma HA levels (median value = 103 µg/l) and serum Ir F-SC levels (median value = 552 ng/ml) were significantly higher than those measured in patients with uncomplicated post-operative evolution (48 µg/l and 200 ng/ml respectively). HA and Ir F-SC concentrations were correlated to the degree of histological abnormalities of endothelial cells and cholangiocytes respectively. Peak of plasma HA levels was observed within the 48 hours before the histological diagnosis of rejection. HA levels were not significantly different in patients with acute rejection and in infected patients, whereas, in this population of transplant patients, Ir F-SC levels were significantly higher in acute rejection than in infection. Treatment of the episode of acute rejection was followed by a rapid decrease of HA levels (2 to 5 days) and a slower decrease of Ir F-SC concentrations (within 30 days). This preliminary study suggests that circulating HA and Ir F-SC levels could be complementary markers of graft rejection after liver transplantation.

Acute allograft rejection is one of the most common causes of hepatic dysfunction after liver transplantation (LT), and up to now, the diagnosis of acute rejection remains difficult. Indeed, clinical and biological signs of acute rejection (AR) are not accurate because of their lack of specificity, and the liver biopsy is necessary to confirm the diagnosis of AR. Typically, histological diagnosis of AR is based on the presence of three pathological features : portal tract inflammatory infiltrate, endothelialitis, and small bile ducts damage. However, the liver biopsy is an invasive method. Moreover, its interpretation is often difficult : histological signs of AR are observed in 2/3 of the transplant patients at the end of the first week (KEMNITZ et al., 1989 ; STARZL et al., 1989 a), even if clinical or biological modifications are lacking. The diagnosis of AR is commonly made after exclusion of other causes of graft dysfunction. So, better diagnosis tools, reflecting the histological targets of AR would be welcome (PAINTAUD & MIGUET, 1991) (Table 1). Hyaluronic acid (HA), a glycosaminoglycan synthetised by the mesenchymal cells, is rapidly cleared from serum and broken down by the liver endothelial cells. High values of HA are correlated with hepatic endothelial cell damage, particularly in liver AR (ADAMS et al., 1989). The immunoreactive free secretory component (Ir F-SC), a glycoprotein belonging to the secretory immunoglobulin structure, is synthetised by the glandular and mucous epithelial cells, and in humans, by biliary epithelial cells. An increase in serum Ir F-SC has been observed in hepatic cholestatic diseases (VUITTON et al., 1991). The aim of this study was to evaluate the interest of plasma HA and serum Ir F-SC serum Ir F-SC levels in AR diagnosis, reflecting *a priori* lesions of the two main immunological targets of AR in the liver.

TABLEAU 1 : NON-CONVENTIONAL TESTS KNOWN TO BE USEFUL IN THE DIGANOSIS OF LIVER ALLOGRAFT REJECTION

IMMUNOLOGICAL MARKERS :		MARKERS OF BILIARY AND ENDOTHELIAL DAMAGE :	
▲ Neopterin		▲ Secretory component	
→ serum	OLDHAFER et al., 88	→ bile	ADAMS et al., 87b
→ urine	TILG et al., 89	→ serum	BRESSON-HADNI et al, 88
▲ Bile chemotactic factors	ADAMS et al., 87a	▲ Hyaluronic Acid	ADAMS et al., 89b POLLARD et al., 90
▲ SIL2-receptor			
→ serum	PERKINS et al., 89		
→ bile, bile/serum	ADAMS et al., 89a		
▲ IL1, IFN , TNF	ADAMS et al., 90 TILG et al., 90		
▲ ß2 microglobulin			
→ bile, bile/serum	ADAMS et al., 87b, 88		
→ serum	TILG et al., 90		
▲ Soluble Class I antigen			
→ bile	POLLARD et al., 89		

PATIENTS AND METHODS :

Fifteen patients were consecutively studied (10 men and 5 women) ; the mean age was 52 (range 39 to 62). Indications for LT were cirrhosis in 6 cases, hepatocellular carcinomas in 7 cases, and primary biliary cirrhosis in 2 cases. Retransplantations, emergency LT, and multiorgan transplantations were excluded. Blood HA and Ir F-SC were determined every day from the first post-operative day to the discharge of the patients. Plasmatic HA was measured by using a sensitive radiometric assay (Pharmacia HA test). An ELISA test was used to measure the serum levels of Ir F-SC as previously described (VINCENT & REVILLARD, 1988). Patients follow-up included daily clinical examination and hepatic blood tests, a weekly ultra-sound and doppler examination of the liver, and a T-tube cholangiography at day 7. A liver biopsy was systematically performed at the 10th day and at any time if clinically indicated. The immunosuppressive regimen associated methylprednisolone, azathioprine and cyclosporine A. In 2 patients with post-operative renal failure, antithymocyte globulins were temporarily prescribed instead of cyclosporine A. For the diagnosis of AR, the criteria used were : increase of conjugated bilirubine, alkaline phosphatases, gammaglutamyl transpeptidase, ALT and AST and a compatible histological pattern of AR. Each of the 3 typicall histological features of AR was scored semi-quantitatively on a scale of 0-3 (0 = absent ; 1 = mild ; 2 = moderate ; 3 = severe) to give a final score of 0-9. A final score of greater than 4 was considered to indicate significant acute rejection. Statistical analyses were performed using Mann Whitney U test, and the Spearman rank correlation.

RESULTS

At the time of AR diagnosis (4 days before and after the first liver biopsy), plasma HA levels (median value = 103 µg/l) were significantly higher in patients with AR, than that in stable patients (median value = 48 µg/l) (fig. I). HA plasma levels were correlated to the degree of histological abnormalities of endothelial cells. However, the highest value of HA was disclosed in infected patients, but in these patients, the median value (= 116 µg/l) was not significantly different from that observed in AR patients.

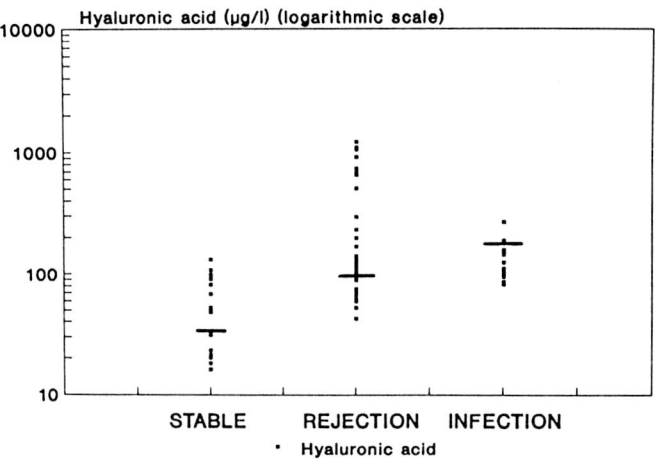

Fig. I : PLASMA CONCENTRATIONS OF HYALURONIC ACID IN 15 PATIENTS AT THE FIRST LIVER BIOPSY (bars represent median values).

In patients with AR, the highest plasma HA levels were observed 48 hours before the histological diagnosis of rejection (Fig. II). Indeed, the return of plasma HA levels to normal values was achieved within only 2 to 5 days. In addition, 48 hours before the first liver biopsy, the HA median value in patients with AR was higher than that measured in stable or infected patients.

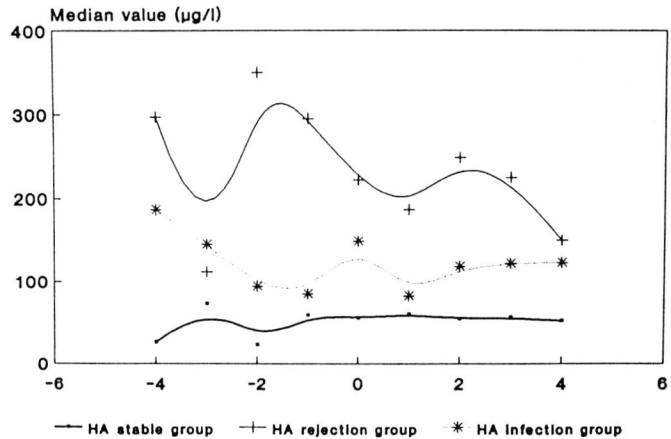

Fig. II : COURSE OF HYALURONIC ACID PLASMA LEVELS FROM DAY-4 TO DAY+4 OF THE FIRST LIVER BIOPSY (day 0 = first liver biopsy)

At the time of AR (4 days before and after the first liver biopsy), the median value of Ir F-SC in AR patients (= 552 ng/ml) was significantly higher than that observed in stable patients (median value = 200 ng/ml) and in infected patients (median value = 179 ng/ml) (Fig. III).

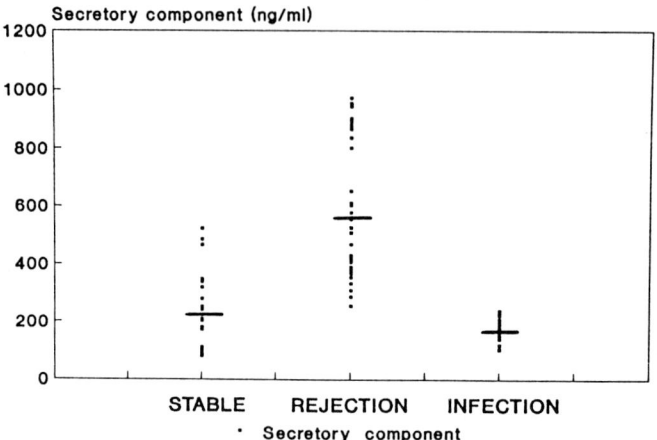

Fig. III : SERUM CONCENTRATIONS OF FREE SECRETORY COMPONENT IN 15 PATIENTS AT THE FIRST LIVER BIOPSY (Bars represent median values).

Ir F-SC serum concentrations were also correlated to the degree of histological lesions of the biliary epithelial cells. Unlike the HA results, the evolution of Ir F-SC in each group of patients remained stable before and after the first liver biopsy. In cases of AR, serum Ir F-SC levels were immediately maximal (as early as 4 days before the liver biopsy) (fig. IV) and remained unchanged during the entire episode of rejection.

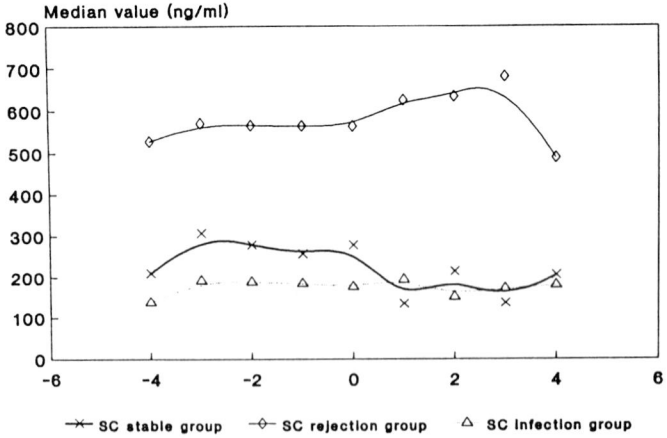

Fig. IV : COURSE OF FREE SECRETORY COMPONENT SERUM LEVELS FROM DAY-4 TO DAY+4 (day 0 = first liver biopsy).

DISCUSSION

Our results suggest that the increase of HA and Ir F-SC during AR reflects the damage of the 2 main targets of AR, entothelial cells and biliary epithelial cells respectively. The long serum half-life of Ir F-SC unlike that of HA could explain the persistance of high serum Ir F-SC levels after the diagnosis of AR. Moreover, the regeneration of cholangiocytes is slower than endothelial cell recovery and this could account for the prolonged increase in serum Ir F-SC.

Our results confirm previous report in liver AR (ADAMS et al., 1989b, BRESSON-HADNI, et al., 1991). However, contrary to the conclusion of ADAMS et al. (1989b), infected patients had high levels of plasma HA and it was not possible to discriminate these patients from those with AR. Interestingly, POLLARD et al. (1989) also disclosed high values of HA in patients who had both rejection and sepsis. It has been demonstrated that HA synthesis could be enhanced by interleukin-1 and interferons (ENGSTRÖM-LAURENT & HÅLLGREN, 1985). Such cytokines are increased during septicaemias, and could explain the HA increase during severe infection. The study of BRESSON-HADNI et al. (1991) indicated that serum Ir F-SC increased during AR but also under other conditions, particularly in infected patients. However, the Ir F-SC bile/serum ratios were significantly higher in patients with AR than in infected patients. In our study, serum Ir F-SC determinations were helpful to discriminate infected patients from patients with AR. These preliminary results suggest that HA and Ir F-SC could be two complementary markers of AR after liver transplantation.

REFERENCES

ADAMS, D.H., BURNETT, D., STOCKLEY, R.A., ELIAS, E. (1987 a) : Leucocyte chemotactic activity in bile during rejection of liver allografts. *J. Hepatol.* 5 (suppl. 1) : S3.

ADAMS, D.H., BURNETT, D., STOCKLEY, R.A., Mac MASTER, P., ELIAS, E. (1987 b) : Markers of biliary epithelial damage in liver allograft rejection. *Transpl. Proc.* 5, 3820-3821.

ADAMS, D.H., BURNETT, D., STOCKLEY, R.A., HUBSCHER, S.G., Mac MASTER P., ELWYN, E. (1988) : Biliary ß2-microglobulin in liver allograft rejection. *Hepatology* 6, 1565-1570.

ADAMS, D.H., WANG, L., HUBSCHER, S.G., ELIAS, E. NEUBERGER, J.M. (1989 a) : Soluble interkin 2 receptors in serum and bile of liver transplant recipients. Lancet 1, 469-471.

ADAMS, D.H., WANG, L., HUBSCHER, S.G., NEUBERGER, J.M. (1989 b) : Hepatic endothelial cells. Targets in liver allograft rejection ? *Transplantation* 47, 479-482.

ADAMS, D.H., GARNER, C., NEUBERGER, J.M. (1990) : Serum tumour necrosis factor alpha in patients following liver transplantation (summary). IV Congress of the European Society for Organ Transplantation. Barcelona, 1-4 novembre, 229.

BRESSON-HADNI, S., SEILLES, E., ROSSEL, M., PARROT, A., CARBILLET, J.P., REVILLARD, J.P., MIGUET, J.P., GILLET, M., VUITTON, D.A. (1988) : La composante sécrétoire des immunoglobulines polymères, nouveau marqueur du rejet de greffe de foie ? Ann. Chir. 42, 692.

BRESSON-HADNI, S., ROSSEL, M., SEILLES, E., VUITTON, D.A., GUENNOUNE, K., HORY, B., MIGUET, J.P., GILLET, M., VINCENT, C., REVILLARD, J.P. (1991) : Serum and bile secretory immunoglobulins and secretory component during the early postoperative course following liver transplantation. *Hepatology* (in press).

ENGSTRÖM-LAURENT, A., & HÄLLGREN, R. (1985) : Circulating hyaluronate in rheumatoid arthritis : relationship to inflammatory activity and the effect of corticosteroid therapy. *Ann. Rheum. Dis.* 44, 83-88.

KEMNITZ, J., GUBERNATIS, G., BUNZENDAHL, H., RINGE, B., PICHLMAYR, R., GEORGII, A. (1989) : Criteria for the histopathological classification of the liver allograft rejection and their clinical relevance. *Transplant. Proc.* 21, 2208-2210.

OLDHAFER, K.J., SCHAEFER, O., WONIGEIT, K., RINGE, B., PICHLAMYR, R. (1988) : Monitoring of serum neopterin levels after liver transplantation. *Transplant Proc* 20, 671-673.

PAINTAUD, G., & MIGUET, J.P. (1991) : Diagnostic tools in liver allograft rejection. *J of Hepatol.* 12, 256-260.

PERKINS, J.D., NELSON, D.L., RAKELA, J., GRAMBSCH, P.M., KROM, R.A.F. (1989) : Soluble interleukin-2 receptor levels as an indicator of liver allograft rejection. *Transplantation* 47, 77-81.

POLLARD, S.G., DAVIES, H.S., CALNE, R.Y. (1989) : Soluble class I antigen in human bile. Transplantation 48, 712-713.

POLLARD, S.G., FORBES, M.A., METCALFE, S.M., COOPER, E.H., CALNE R.Y. (1990) : Hyaluronic acid in the assessment of liver graft function. *Transplant Proc* 22, 2301-2302.

STARZL, T.E., DEMETRIS, A.J. & VAN THIEL, D. (1989 a) : Liver transplantation. *N Eng J Med* 321, 1092-1097.

STARZL, T.E., TODO, S., TZAKIS, A.G., GORDON, R.D., MAKOWKA, L., STIEBER, A., PODESTA L., YANAGA, K., CONCEPCION, W., IWATSUKI, S. (1989 b) : Liver transplantation : an unfinished product. *Transplant Proc* 21, 2197-2200.

TILG, H., VOGEL, N., AULITZKY, W.E., SCHÖNITZER, D., MARGREITER, R., DIETZE, O., JUDMAIER, G., WACHTER, H., HUBER, C. (1989) : Neopterin excretion after liver transplantation and its value in differential diagnosis of complications. *Transplantation* 48, 594-599.

TILG, H., VOGEL, N., AULITZKY, W.E., HEROLD, M., KÖNIGSRAINEN, A., MARGREITER, R., HUBER, C. (1990) : Evaluation of cytokines and cytokine induced secondary messages in sera of patients after liver transplantation. *Transplantation* 49, 1074-1080.

VINCENT, C., REVILLARD, J.P. (1988) : Sandwich-type ELISA for free and bound secretory component in human biological fluids. *J. Immunol. Methods* 106, 153-160.

VUITTON, D.A., SEILLES, E., COZON, G., ROSSEL, M., BRESSON-HADNI, S., REVILLARD, J.P. (1991) : Secretory Immunoglobulin A in hepatobiliary diseases. *Surv. Dig. Dis.* 9, 78-91.

Immunological, metabolic and infectious aspects of liver transplantation. Eds D.A. Vuitton, C. Balabaud, D. Houssin, D. Dhumeaux. John Libbey Eurotext, Paris © 1991, pp. 65-75.

Prevention of hepatitis B virus (HBV) recurrence in liver transplant recipients by passive immunization

Rainer Müller, Gundolf Gubernatis, Margarete Farle, Gabrielle Niehoff, Heide Klein, Christian Wittekind, Günter Tusch, Hans-Ulrich Lautz, Klaus Böker, Walter Stangel, Rudolf Pichlmayr

Abteilung für Gastroenterologie und Hepatologie, Klinik für Abdominal und Transplantations-chirurgie, Institut für Pathologie, Abteilung für Immunologie und Transfusions-medizin, Medizinische Hochschule Hannover, Germany
Address for correspondence : Abteilung für Gastroenterologie und Hepatologie, Medizinische Hochschule Hannover, Konstanty-Gutschow-Strasse 8, D-3000 Hannover 61, Germany

Abstract

Liver transplantation in HBs-antigen (HBsAg) positive allograft recipients is associated with a high risk of HBV recurrence sometime after surgery. So far, the results of measures to prevent recurrent HBV-infection by means of treatment with interferon, hepatitis B vaccination and short-term passive immunization with hepatitis B immunoglobuline (HBIg) or monoclonal antibody to HBsAg (anti-HBs) were disappointing. In the present study the results of long-term, anti-HBs monitored passive immunization with HBIg is reported. In 23 HBsAg positive liver transplant recipients an anti-HBs level of ≥100 IU/l was maintained for six months or for 12 months respectively. The rate of recurrent infection was found less than 20% under HBIg substitution, whereas 11 graft recipients without any or short term HBIg prophylaxis were reinfected by month 15 after transplantation. HBV-recurrence was associated with a high mortality rate, chronic liver disease and recurrent cirrhosis in the allograft.

Key words:
Hepatitis B, liver transplantation, hepatitis B immunoglobuline prophylaxis.

Introduction

Liver transplantation in the presence of circulating HBsAg entails a serious risk for HBV infection of the hepatic allograft. Still limited experience today indicates that the infection will recur in the vast majority of HBsAg positive liver graft recipients (Gordon et al. 1986, Demetris et al. 1986, Portmann et al. 1986, Carey et al. 1988, Iwatsuki et al. 1988). Various attempts to prevent recurrence of infection including treatment with interferons, hepatitis B vaccination and short term passive immunization with polyclonal HBIg or monoclonal anti-HBs have been discouraging.

Human interferons have been shown to suppress HBV replication and treatment with interferon alpha has proven beneficial in patients with chronic hepatitis B and persistent viremia. However therapy with interferon in immunocompromised patients is less effective. So far, interferon treatment for prevention of recurrent HBV infection after transplantation was not sucessful (Rakela et al. 1989). Furthermore interferon treatment might give rise to the fear to promote the risk of rejection, as the expression of HLA class I antigens on cell surfaces is enhanced after exposure to interferon (Manabe et al. 1986, Pignatelli et al. 1986).

Plasma-derived and recombinant HBsAg particles vaccines have proven highly immunogenic and efficacious in preventing hepatitis B among healthy adult populations at risk of HBV-infection, but vaccine immunogenicity in immunocompromised patients is still found low. This also appears to be the case for liver graft recipients. Hepatitis B vaccination with "pre-s" and "s" containing antigens has failed to induce an anti-H- response in vaccinees after tansplantation (Rizzetto et al. 1987). However, protective anti-HBs serum levels for prevention of hepatitis B after accidental needle stick exposure may be attained passively by administration of hepatitis B immunoglobulin. Early experience with either polyclonal HBIg or high-titer monoclonal anti-HBs in a small number of HBsAg positive liver transplant recipients appeared to be promising (Ferla et al. 1988, Müller et al. 1988, Colledan et al. 1989, Reynes et al. 1989, Starzl et al. 1989). In the present study we report the outcome of HBsAg positive liver transplant recipients after long-term postsurgical HBIg prophylaxis.

Patients

The course of 34 HBsAg positive liver transplant recipients, 29 males and five females, aged from 13 to 62 (mean 38 years old) was evaluated. Indication for liver grafting were hepato-cirrhosis in 19 patients, hepatocellular carcinoma in 12 patients, fulminant liver failure in two individuals and a Budd-Chiari Syndrom in one patient. Besides HBsAg the preoperative serological HBV marker profiles revealed HBV-DNA and HBeAg in four patients, HBeAg without presence of HBV-DNA in 10 patients, HBV-DNA and anti-HBe in two patients, anti-HBe without HBV-DNA in 12 patients and neither HBV-DNA nor HBeAg nor anti-HBe in six patients.

Methods

Liver function tests and HBV serology were performed according to standard methods. The anti-HBs concentrations in the serum were calculated by using the formula specified by Hollinger (1982). The monitoring for anti-HBs serum concentrations was performed once per month after transplantation. HBV-DNA was demonstrated by the Hep Probe™ (GIBCO/BRL, Life Technologies Eggenstein-Leopoldshafen, West Germany). The numerical score described by Knodell (1981) was applied for evaluation of liver histopathology.

Hepatitis B immunologuline prophylaxis

A polyvalent HBIg preparation obtained from anti-delta-negative donor sera after native HBV infection (Hepatect^R Biotest Ltd., Frankfurt/Main, West Germany) was used for passive immunization. The anti-HBs content was 50 IU/ml. HBIg was administered intravenously according to three different schedules.

Six patients received HBIg only in the anhepatic phase during surgery. The doses administered varied between 2,400 IU and 128,000 IU (x 32,000 IU) of anti-HBs.

In 11 liver graft recipients HBIg treatment with 10,000 IU anti-HBs was started in the anhepatic phase. The same dose was administered every day for the first eight days after transplantation. Further HBIg substitution with 10,000 IU anti-HBs was continued according to the anti-HBs blood level. An anti-HBs level of at least 100 IU/l in the serum was maintained for six months.

Another 12 individuals received HBIg according to the same schedule as that applied in the previous group of 11 patients apart from two modifications: anti-HBs blood level of ≥100 IU/l were maintained for 12 months and 40,000 IU anti-HBs per day were given to HBV-DNA-positive transplant recipience for the first eight days after operation.

No HBIg prophylaxis was performed in five HBsAg positive liver transplant patients.

Results

The proportion of recurrent HBV infections in the various series of investigations is shown in Figure 1. HBV recurrence rates under long-term substitution of HBIg with anti-HBs maintenace levels of ≥100 IU/l were found 18% and 25% respectively after six months or 12 months of prophylaxis. In both groups, the frequency of recurrent infections increased after discontinuation of HBIg administration. Twenty-four months after transplantation, the sera of three out of nine patients were still found to be negative for HBsAg. It may be assumed that they have definitively elliminated the virion.

All patients who had not received any passive immunization or in whom HBIg was only administered during the anhepatic phase of surgery, experienced recurrent HBV infection within one to 15 months after transplantation.

The preoperative HBV marker profile in the serum is a crucial indicator for HBV recurrence. Apart from one exception, HBV infection recured in all inviduals in whom HBV-DNA and/or HBeAg was preoperatively demonstrated in the serum.

The clinical significance of recurrent HBV infection after liver transplantation was analysed of the basis of the mortality, the results of liver function tests and the findings of liver histopathology. Out of the 34 patients evaluated, nine had died. All of them belonged to the group of 23 patients with HBV recurrence (39%).

Reappearance of HBsAg was associated with a significant rise of aminotransferase activities in the serum. None of the patients cleared the HBsAg during follow-up. All developed a persistent HBs antigenemia. The mean enzyme activities differed significantly from those of the transplant recipients without

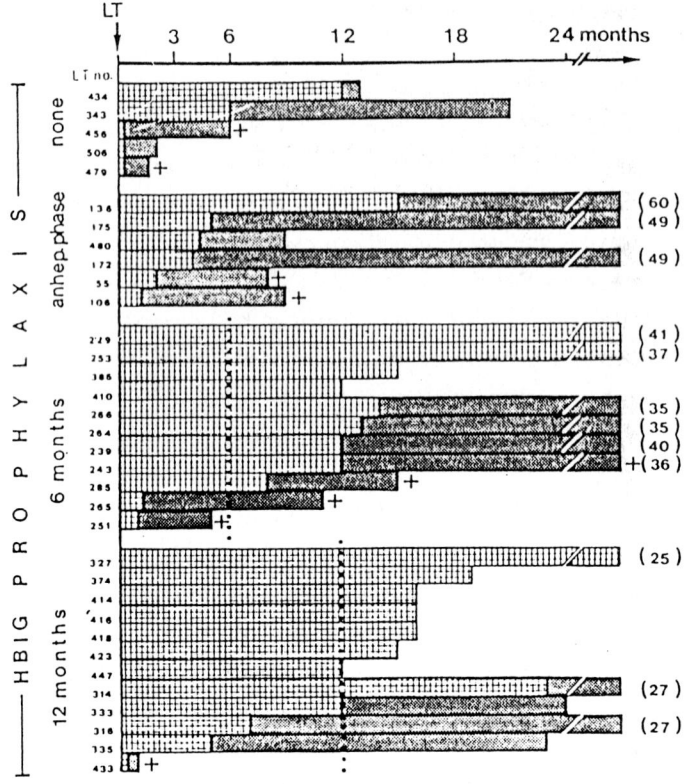

Figure 1
HBsAg recurrence after liver transplantation (LT) in the various series of investigations.

Symbols: ▦ serum HBsAg-negative
            ▨ serum HBsAg-positive
          : end of HBIg prophylaxis
         ( ) months after transplantation
          + deceased

HBV recurrence. Activities remained elevated above the normal range, indicating chronic liver disease.

The histological examination of the last follow-up biopsies available in eight patients with HBV recurrence revealed "acute hepatitis" in one individual, "chronic persistent hepatitis" in two subjects, "chronic aggressive hepatitis" in three patients and "liver cirrhosis" in two patients. The results are shown in Figure 2. On the other hand, five biopsies taken from five patients without recurrent infection five to 24 months after transplantation showed nonspecific hepatic lesions without histological signs of chronic hepatitis.

Conclusions

Long-term HBIg prophylaxis with maintenance anti-HBs serum levels of at least 100 IU/l provides an effective measure for prevention of HBV recurrence in liver transplant recipients with a low replicative state of HBV. However recurrence of the infection may occur after discontinuation of HBIg substitution even for over 12 months. Reinfection after such a long period might be attributed to virus particles deriving from extra-hepatic replication (Zignego et al. 1988). Extrachromosomal HBV-DNA, transcripts, translation products such as HBsAg and HBcAg and virion-like Dane particles have been detected in non-hepatic tissues (Romet-Lemonne et al. 1983, Elfassi et al. 1984, Colucci et al. 1988).

Prevention of HBV recurrence with long-term HBIg treatment in HBV-DNA positive liver graft recipients was unsuccessfull. The postsurgical management for this group of transplant patients still remains unresolved.

After transplantation recurrent at hepatitis B was usually found to be anicteric with AST levels which were less than

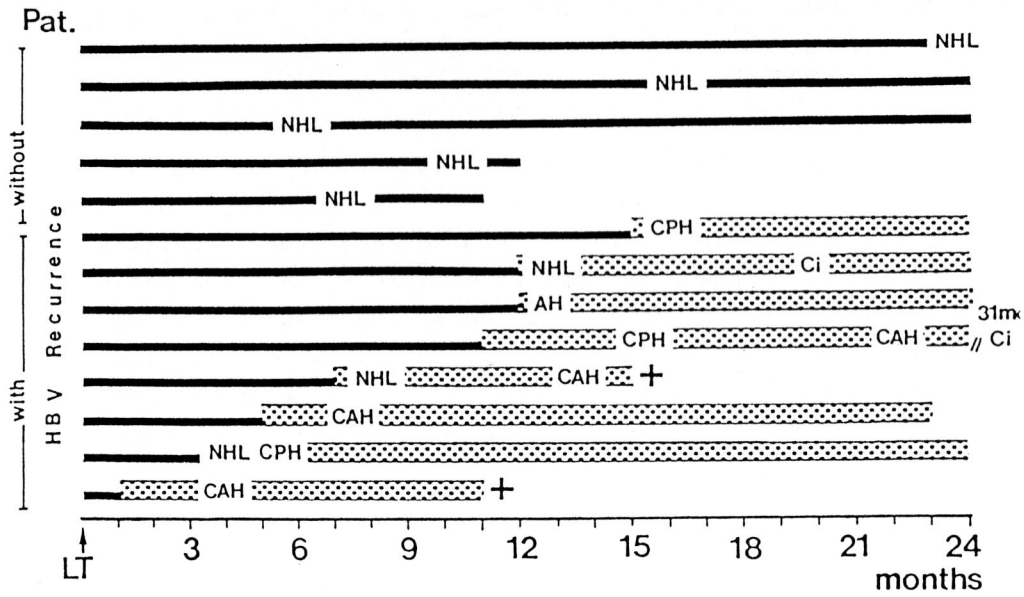

Figure 2
Histological findings of 13 HBsAg-positive liver transplant recipients with and without HBV recurrence.

Symbols:

AH = acute hepatitis
NHL = nonspecific hepatic lesions
CPH = chronic persistent hepatitis
CAH = chronic aggressive hepatitis
CI = cirrhosis

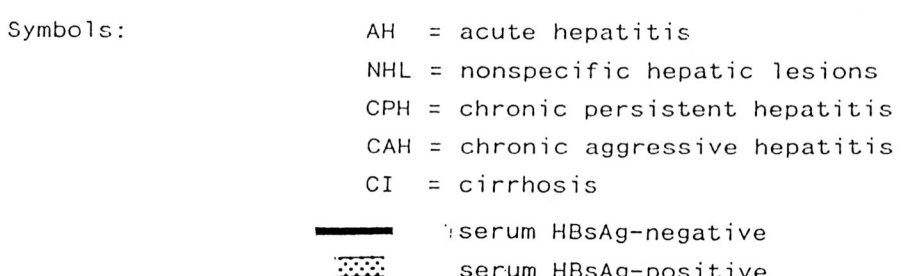

—— serum HBsAg-negative
▒▒▒ serum HBsAg-positive

twice normal. Despite this mild subclinical picture the disease usually runs a chronic course, and chronic agressive hepatitis on biopsy with recurrent cirrhosis may occur.

On the basis of these findings, the indication for liver transplantation in HBsAg-positive recipients is crucially associated with a treatment procedure for successful prevention of recurrent HBV infection in the hepatic allograft after surgery.

This study was supported by the Deutsche Forschungsgemeinschaft, Forschergruppe Organtransplantation, Project A5.

References

1. Carey WD, Tuthill R, Winkelman E, Vogt D., Broughan T. (1988): Clinical and pathological sequelae of orthotopic liver transplantation in chronic B hepatitis. In Zuckerman, A.J. (ed):"Viral Hepatitis and Liver Disease." New York: Alan R.Liss, pp 801-807.

2. Colledan M, Grendele M, Gridelli B, Rossi G, Fassati LR, Ferla G, Doglia M, Gislon M, Galmarini D (1989): Long-term results after liver transplantation in B and delta hepatitis. Transplantation Proceedings 21:2421-2423.

3. Colucci G, Lyons P, Beazer Y, Waksal SD (1988): Production of hepatitis B virus-infected human B-cell hybridomas: transmission of the viral genome to normal lymphocytes in cocultures. Virology 164:238-244.

4. Demetris AJ, Jaffe R, Sheahan DG, Burham J, Spero J, Iwatsuki S, van Thiel DH, Starzl TE (1986): Recurrent hepatitis B in liver allograft recipients: differentiation between viral hepatitis B and rejection. American Journal of Pathology 125: 161-172.

5. Elfassi E, Romet-Lemonne JL, Essex M, Frances-McLane MF, Haseltine WA (1984): Evidence of extrachromosomal forms of hepatitis B viral DNA in a bone marrow culture obtained from a patient recently infected with hepatitis B virus. Proceedings of the National Academy of Science, USA 81:3526-3528.

6. Ferla G, Colledan M, Doglia M, Fassati LR, Gislon M, Gridelli B, Rossi G, Galmarini D (1988): B hepatitis and liver transplantation. Transplantation Proceedings 20: Suppl.1, 566-569.

7. Gordon RD, Shaw BW Jr, Iwatsuki S, Esquivel CO, Starzl TE (1986): Indications for liver transplantation in the cyclosporine era. Surgery Clinical North America 66: 541-556.

8. Hollinger FB, Adam E, Heiberg D, Melnick JL (1982): Response to hepatitis B vaccine in a young adult population. In Szmuness W, Alter HJ, Maynard JE, (eds): "Viral Hepatitis" 1981 International Symposium, Philadelphia PA: Franklin Inst Press, pp 451-466.

9. Iwatsuki S, Starzl TE, Todo S, Gordon RD, Esquivel CO, Tzakis AG, Makowka L, Marsh JW, Koneru B, Stieber A, Klintmalm G, Husberg B (1988): Experience in 1000 liver transplants under cyclosporine-steroid therapy: a survival report. Transplantation Proceedings 20 (Suppl.1): 498-504.

10. Knodell RG, Ishak KG, Black WC, Chen TS, Craig RC, Kaplowitz N, Kiernan TW, Woilman J (1981): Formulation and application of a numerical scoring system for assessing histological activity in asymptomatic chronic active hepatitis. Hepatology 1:431-435.

11. Manabe K, Yamada G, Nagashima H (1986): Immunohisto chemical study of HLA class I antigens on the hepatocytes of patients with chronic hepatitis B. Gastroenterology Japan 21:357-364.

12. Müller R, Lauchart W, Farle M, Klein H, Niehoff G, Pichlmayr R. (1988): Simultaneous passive-active immunization for preventing hepatitis B virus reinfection in hepatitis B surface antigen-positive liver transplant recipients. In: A.J. Zuckermann (ed): " Viral Hepatitis and Liver Disease." New York: Alan R. Liss, Incorporation, pp 810-812.

13. Pignatelli M, Waters J, Brown D, Lever A, Iwarson S, Schaff Z, Gerety R, Thomas HC (1986): HLA class I antigens on the hepatocyte membrane during recovery from acute hepatitis B virus infection and during interferon therapy in chronic hepatitis B virus infection. Hepatology 6:349-353.

14. Portmann B, O'Grady J, Williams R (1986): Disease recurrence following orthotopic liver transplantation. Transplantation Proceedings 18 (Suppl.4): 136-143.

15. Rakela J, Woofen R, Batts KP, Perkins JD, Taswell HF, Krom RAF (1989): Failure of interferon to prevent recurrent hepatitis B infection in hepatic allograft. Mayo Clinic Proceedings 64:429-432.

16. Rakela J (1989): Recurrent hepatitis B infection in hepatic allograft. Mayo Clinic Proceedings 64:597.

17. Reynès M, Zignego L, Fabiani SB, Gugenheim J, Tricottet V, Bréchot C, Bismuth H (1989): Graft hepatitis delta virus reinfection after orthotopic liver transplantation in HDV cirrhosis. Transplantation Proceedings 21:2424-2425.

18. Rizzetto M, Macagno S, Chiaberge E, Verme G, Negro F, Marinueci G, di Giacomo C, Alfani D, Cortesini R, Milazzo F, Dogeia M, Fassati LR, Galmarini D (1987): Liver transplantation in hepatitis delta virus disease. Lancet II:469-471.

19. Romet-Lemorine JL, McLane MF, Elfassi E, Haseltine WA, Azocar J, Essex M (1983): Hepatitis B virus infection in cultured human lymphoblastoid cells. Science 221:667-669.

20. Starzl TE, Todo S, Tzakis AG, Gordon RD, Makowka L, Stieber A, Podesta L, Yanaga K (1989): Liver transplantation: An unfinished product. Transplantation Proceedings 21 (1Pt2): 2197-2200.

21. Torisu M, Yokoyama T, Amemiya H, Kohler PF, Schroter G, Martinean G, Penn I, Palmer W, Halgrimson CG, Putnam CW, Starzl TE (1971): Immunosuppression, liver injury, and hepatitis in renal, hepatic, and cardiac homograft recipients. Annals of Surgery 174:620-637.

22. Zignego AL, Samuel D, Gugenheim J, Chardan B, Bismuth A, Hadchouel M, Reynes M, Bréchot C, Bismuth H (1988): Hepatitis B virus replication and mononuclear blood cell infection after liver transplantation. In Zuckerman AJ (ed): Viral Hepatitis and Liver Disease. New York: Alan R.Liss, pp 808-809.

Immunological, metabolic and infectious aspects of liver transplantation. Eds D.A. Vuitton, C. Balabaud, D. Houssin, D. Dhumeaux. John Libbey Eurotext, Paris © 1991, pp. 77-81.

Incidence and prognosis of viral infections due to herpes viruses (other than cytomegalovirus), adenoviruses and hepatitis C virus in liver transplant recipients

Elisabeth Dussaix

Laboratoire de Virologie, Hôpital de Bicêtre, 94275, Le Kremlin-Bicêtre Cedex, France

Viral infections remain a significant cause of morbidity and mortality in liver transplant recipients. Cytomegalovirus is considered as the most common etiologic viral pathogen but the other members of the herpes group (herpes simplex virus, varicella-zoster virus, Epstein-Barr virus, human herpes virus-6), the adenoviruses and the hepatitis C virus can also induce unfavorable infectious complications. Most of these viruses can remain in a latent state within the host and can be reactivated by the immunosuppressive therapy or by the allogenic contact between graft an host. Further, latent viruses can be transmitted by blood transfusions or transplanted livers from seropositive donor to seronegative recipients.

HERPES SIMPLEX VIRUS INFECTIONS

Symptomatic Herpes simplex virus (HSV) infections are frequent in liver recipients, occuring in over 35% of patients within the first month following the transplantation (Breinig et al, 1987; Singh et al, 1988). Most cases are the result of latent virus reactivation. The transmission of HSV by the donor organ which has been documented for renal and heart recipients (Goodman, 1989) is rare but also possible in liver recipients (Singh etal, 1988). The majority of patients develop typical oral or genital mucocutaneous HSV lesions which usually heal spontaneously or after acyclovir therapy. Oesophagitis or severe perianal ulcerations with proctitis can be observed. In contrast, visceral (hepatitis, pneumopathy, encephalitis) or disseminated HSV infections are uncommon.

VARICELLA-ZOSTER VIRUS INFECTIONS

Less than 10% of adult liver recipients develop clinical varicella-zoster virus (VZV) infections during the months or years following the transplantation (Singh et al, 1988). Ninety eight percent of them are localised dermatomal zoster, however cutaneous dissemination of vesicles to sites distant from the involved dermatome can be seen. The central nervous system may be also involved. Varicella is more frequent in pediatric liver recipients (Breinig et al 1988). The spectrum of illness is broad including mild infections and serious diseases. Nevertheless the incidence of these latter are more frequent. In many cases, the lesions are bullous or hemorragic with pulmonary involvement. Encephalitis, cerebellar ataxia can be observed. Zoster and varicella improve usually after acyclovir treatment but, despite of this, fatal disseminated varicella can still occur. Specific anti VZV globulins (VZIG) may prevent or attenuate the illness in patients without a previous history of chickenpox or in those known to be seronegative for VZV. The efficacity of VZIG treatment depends on the precocious administration within 72 h of exposure.

EPSTEIN-BARR VIRUS INFECTIONS

Epstein-Barr virus (EBV) infections are also frequent in liver recipients since 30 to 60% of them have serologic evidence of active disease during the first six months following the transplantation (Breinig et al.; Singh et al, 1988; Randhawa et al, 1990) The incidence of EBV infections is, however, higher in pediatric (57%) than in adult (24 to 36%) populations.
Sixty seven to 82% of patients who are seronegative for EBV before transplantation develop primary EBV infection after transplantation. Most cases are asymptomatic. Clinical manifestations can be those of classic infectious mononucleosis but pulmonary involvement is frequently observed in children. In some cases, the symptomatology do not differ from that of CMV infection. Thirty to 50% of recipients who are seropositive for EBV before transplantation present with viral reactivation which is also often asymptomatic, however a wide variety of syndrome related to EBV infection can be seen. Clinical EBV manifestations improve usually spontaneously or after a reduction of immunosuppression and a course of acyclovir. One to 4% of liver recipients, especially those who experience a primary EBV infection, develop uncontroled B lymphocyte proliferation which can progress to fatal monoclonal lymphoma. EBV-related lymphoproliferative disease, in its early stages regresses when cyclosporine is discontinued or acyclovir is administered.

HERPES VIRUS 6 INFECTIONS

First described in 1986 as human B lymphotropic virus (Salahuddin et al, 1986), the human herpes virus 6 (HHV-6) is a new herpes virus widespread in general population as judged by the high prevalence of antibody to this agent in healthy adults. Primary HHV-6 infection occurs usually in early life. In some cases, it is associated to exanthem subitum, a common febrile illness with rash in childhood (Yamananishi et al, 1988). However, the asymptomatic infection seems to be more frequent. In vitro, the virus shows a tropism for CD4 + T cells but it can infect a variety of other cell types including B cells, glial cells, mononuclear cells and megacaryocytes (Lusso et al, 1987). In vivo, it was originally isolated from blood of patients with acquired immunodeficiency syndrome and other hematologic disorders. It was also isolated from the peripheral blood lymphocytes of children with exanthem subitum and more recently from the saliva of healthy adults (Harnett et al, 1990).
A fatal case of fulminant hepatitis, associated with HHV-6 infection was reported in a 3 month-old boy (Yoshizo et al, 1990). The virus was isolated from peripheral blood mononuclear cells and HHV-6 gene

sequence was found in brain and liver tissues. Transient raised serum transaminase activity have been described in two immunocompetent adults (Niederman et al, 1988) and in a 2 month-old infant with HHV-6 infection (Tajirih et al 1990). Further, acute HHV-6 infection with deterioration of liver functions was observed in a seronegative for HHV-6 patient 15 days after liver transplantation from a donor seropositive for HHV-6 (Ward et al, 1989). As the other herpes viruses, HHV-6 probably remains latent in the body after primary infection and may be transmitted by liver graft or blood transfusion. This virus could be responsable of some cases of acute hepatitis observed in liver recipients.

ADENOVIRUS INFECTIONS

Adenovirus (AV) infections have been associated, in some instances, with serious infections in immunocompromised patients including renal and bone marrow transplants (Zahradnik et al, 1988). In liver transplant recipients, the incidence of AV infections is well documented only in pediatric recipients (Koneru et al 1987). As estimated by isolation of virus from throat, swab, urine or stool specimens, 8,4% of children who received a liver graft, develop AV infection whithin a post-transplantation period of 5 days to 2 years or later. Clinical symptoms are usually missing or limited to fever, respiratory signs, conjunctivitis or diarrhea. However, fatal invasive infections have been reported by several authors (Koneru et al, 1987; Wreghitt et al, 1989; Varki et al, 1990). These infections occured within an interval of 5 days to 30 days following the transplantation. Most of them included hepatitis which in some cases had been mistakenly treated as a rejection. These cases emphasize the need to perform a liver biopsy whenever allograft dysfunction is detected. In three cases, patients underwent retransplantation but AV hepatitis recured in second allograft of two patients who died of disseminated AV disease.

HEPATITIS C VIRUS

Hepatitis c virus (HCV) is considered as the most frequent transfusion hepatitis-associated viral agent. Liver transplant recipients are at high risk of HCV infection because they often need multiple blood transfusions during surgery. However the true prevalence of HCV posttransplant hepatitis is still difficult to precise. Until recently, the diagnosis of HCV infection was based on the measurement of antibody to the C-100-3 antigen. This recombinant non structural HCV-associated protein was used to coat wells of microtitre trays of the Ortho Diagnostic Systems enzyme-linked-immuno assay (ELISA). Anti C-100-3 antibody appears lastly, between 2 and 6 months even one year after the onset of hepatitis. Thus, some cases of HCV infection can be misdiagnosed if sequential serum samples taken over a prolonged period are not tested. In contrast, false positive results have been reported in patients with hypergammaglobulinemia (McFarlane et al, 1990). Using the first generation ELISA tests, Grendele et al (1990) found that only 8% of liver recipients followed for up at least 6 months and seronegative for HCV before transplantation became anti-HCV antibody positive after transplantation. Two patients had transient hepatitis. Four of 6 patients seropositive for HCV before transplantation, had lost antibody between the 4th and the 10th month after transplantation. The recent incorporation of additional non structural(C-5-1-1,C-33-c) and structural (C-22-3) recombinant HCV proteins has improved not only the assay specificity but also the assay sensitivity for detecting HCV earlier in infection. The avaibility in the near future of these new tests will allow to determine the exact pathogenicity of HCV in liver transplant recipients.

REFERENCES.

Breinig, M.K., Zitelli, B. and Starzl, T.E.(1987):Epstein-Barr virus, cytomegalovirus and other viral infections in children after liver transplantation. J.Infect.Dis.156,273-279.
Goodman, J.L. (1989): possible transmission of herpes simplex virus by organ transplantation.Transplantation, 47,609-613
Grendele, M., Gridelli, B. (1989) : hepatitis C virus infection and liver transplantation. Lancet,ii,1221-1222.
Harnett, G.B., Farr, T.J., Pietroboni, G.R. and Bucens, M.R.(1990) :frequent shedding of human herpes virus-6 in saliva. J. Med. virol.,30, 128-130.
Koneru,B., Jaffe, R.,Esquivel, C.O.,Kunz, R., Todo, S., Iwatsuki, S. and Starzl, T.E.(1987): adenoviral infections in pediatric liver transplant recipients.JAMA, 258, 489-492.
Lusso, P., Salahuddin S.Z.,Ablashi, D.V.,Gallo, R.C., di Marzo Veronese,F.,Markham, P.D. (1987) :diverse tropism of human B lymphotropic virus (human herpes virus-6). Lancet, ii, 743-744.
McFarlane G., Smith ,H.M., Johnson P.J., Bray G.P., Vergani D. and Williams R. (1990): hepatitis C virus antibodies in chronic active hepatitis :pathogenetic factor or false-positive result ? Lancet, i, 754-757
Niederman, J.C., Liu, C.R., Kaplan, M.H., and Brown, N.A. (1988) : clinical and serological features of human herpes virus-6 infection in three adults. Lancet,ii, 817-819.
Randhawa, P.S., Markin R.S., Starzl, T.E. and Demetris, A.J. (1990): Epstein-Barr virus associated syndromes inimmunosuppressed liver transplant recipients. Am. J. Pathol., 14, 538-547.
Salahuddin, S.Z., Ablashi, D.V., Markham,P.D. Josephs, S.F., Sturzenegger, S., Kaplan,M., Halligan, G., Biberfeld, Wong-Staal, F.,Kramarsky B., Gallo, c.(1986) :isolation of a new virus, HBLV, in patient with lymphoproliferative disorders. Science,234, 596-600.
Singh, N., Dummer, J.,Kusne, S., Breinig M.K., Amstrong, T.A. and Makowka, L., and Starzl, T.E., HO, M. (1988): infections with cytomegalovirus and other herpesviruses in 121 liver transplant recipients/ transmission by donated organ and the effect of OK T 3 antibodies. J. Infect. Dis., 158, 124-131.
Tajiri, H., Nose, O., Baba, K. and Okada, S.(1990): human herpes virus-6 infection with liver injury in neonatal hepatitis. Lancet, i, 863.
Varki, N.M., Bhutas, S., Drake, T. and Porter, D.D. (1990): adenovirus hepatitis in two successive liver transplants in child. Arch. Pathol. Lab. Med., 114,106-109.
Ward, K.N., Gray, J.J. and Efstathiou, S. (1989): primary human herpesvirus-6 infection in a patient following liver transplantation from a seropositive donnor.J. Med. Virol., 28, 69-72.
Wreghitt, T.G., Gray, J.J., Ward, K.N., Salt, A., Taylor, D.L., Alp, N.J. and Tyms, A.S.(1989): disseminated adenovirus infection after liver transplantation and its possible treatment with ganciclovir. J.Infect., 19, 88-89.
Yamanishi, K., Toshiomi, O., Sheraki, K., Takahashi,M., Kondo, T., Asano, Y.andKurata, T. (1988): Lancet, i, 1065-1067.

Yoshizo, A., Yoshikawa, T., Suga,S., Yazaki,T, Kondo, K.,and Yamanishi, K.(1990): fatal fulminant hepatitis in an infant with human herpes virus-6 infection. Lancet, i, 862-863.

Zahradnik, J.M., Spencer, M.J. and Porter, D.(1988): adenovirus infection in the immunocompromised patient. Am. J. Med., 68, 725-732.

Lymphoproliferative disorders in organ transplant recipients

Daniel Cherqui

Service de Chirurgie Générale et Digestive, Hôpital Henri Mondor, 94010 Créteil, France

Increased incidence of malignancies in organ transplant recipients was first reported in 1969 (Penn ; McKhann). In 1983, it was estimated that the risk of developing a cancer after an organ transplantation was 100 times higher than in the general population and that of developing a lymphoma 350 times (Hanto et al.). Penn reported recently data from the "Cincinnati Transplant Tumor Registry" including 5250 posttransplant malignancies that occured in 4933 patients (Penn, 1991). These data showed an increased incidence of carcinomas of the skin, vulva, perineum and kidney, hepatobiliary tumors, Kaposi sarcomas and lymphomas. These latter tumors are also called posttransplant lymphoproliferative disorders (PTLDs) and they will be detailed herein.

ROLE OF NEW IMMUNOSUPPRESSIVE REGIMENS

One striking figure of the last decade is the rising proportion of PTLDs among post transplant malignancies. With so-called conventional immunosuppression (azathioprine or cyclophosphamide and prednisone), PTLDs accounted for 11% of post transplant malignancies, but this proportion rose to 26% with cyclosporine A and 64% with monoclonal antibody OKT3 (Penn, 1991). In addition, PTLDs occurred earlier after transplantation with a mean delay of onset of 48, 15 and 7 months, respectively ; 32% and 64% of PTLDs occurred within the first 4 months in the patients treated with cyclosporine A and OKT3, respectively (Penn, 1991).

This phenomenon is probably the result of a more powerful immunosuppression, especially with the use of assocative regimens (Penn, 1991). However, a direct lymphomagenetic effect of OKT3 has been suggested (Swinnen et al., 1990 ; Renard et al.,1991). In a series of heart transplant patients, the rate of PTLDs rose from 1.3% to

11.4% when OKT3 was included to the immunosuppressive regimen in replacement of antithymocyte globulins. In addition, the occurrence of PTLDs was dependant of the cumulative dose of OKT3 with 35.7% of the patients having received a cumulative dose of OKT3 of more than 75 mg who developed PTLD (Swinnen et al., 1990).

ROLE OF THE TRANSPLANTED ORGANS

In one series of patients treated with cyclosporin and steroids between 1979 and 1983, Starzl et al. (1984) reported an incidence of PTLD of 2.5% in renal recipients, 3.5% in liver recipients, 6.3% in heart recipients and 33% in heart-lung recipients. In the most recent series from Pittsburgh (Stieber et al., 1991), 46 of 1276 (3.6%) liver transplant recipients developed PTLD. Among post transplant malignancies of the Cincinnati Registry, 11% were PTLD in renal recipients versus 52% in non renal recipients (Penn, 1991). Recently, two teams independently reported multivisceral transplantations (liver, pancreas and intestine) in four children (Starzl et al., 1989 ; Williams et al., 1989). Immunosuppression included cyclosporin and OKT3 in addition to steroids and azathioprine. Two children died of early postoperative complications and the 2 others of PTLD 3 and 6 months posttransplant.

The different incidence of PTLDs according to the transplanted organs is probably the result of varied levels of immunosuppresion rather than the effect of the organs themselves. Indeed, a more intense immunosuppression is used to save life supporting nonrenal transplants from rejection, whereas renal recipients can return to dialysis (Penn, 1991).

PATHOPHYSIOLOGY OF PTLD : ROLE OF EPSTEIN-BARR VIRUS

Ninety percent of PTLD are due to B lymphocyte proliferation but T-cell or null-cell lymphomas and Hodgkin's diseases have been reported. All types of B lymphocyte proliferations may be seen ranging fron polyclonal to monoclonal. In one series of PTLDs in 46 liver transplant patients, 30% of the proliferations were found to be monoclonal, 40% polyclonal and 30% undetermined (Stieber et al., 1991). Clonality can be explored by cell surface immunoglobulin phenotype but is best explored by gene rearrangement studies using molecular biology (Arnold et al., 1983).

Evidence has been reported that Epstein-Barr virus (EBV) is involved in most (if not all) B-cell proliferations in transplant recipients (Hanto, 1983 ; Ho, 1988). Clinical or serologic signs of EBV infection often herald PTLD. EBV DNA and/or expression of viral proteins have been found in tumor cells. The mechanism of EBV induced B-cell proliferation is well established (Reyes, 1991). EBV is a herpes group virus with a special tropism for B lymphocytes. EBV is a potent polyclonal mitogen for normal B-cells equiped with the CD21 molecule (EBV receptor). B-cells infected by EBV can be cultured in vitro as immortalized lymphoblastoid cell lines. In vivo, EBV infection leads to B cell polyclonal proliferation. After acute EBV infection, latent non lytic infection will remain in most target B-cells with persistence of EBV DNA. B-cell proliferation is prevented by cytotoxic T lymphocyte HLA restricted control. Expression of the Latent Membrane Protein by infected B-cells is thought to account for their recognition by cytotoxic T-cells.

Posttransplant immunosuppression results in iatrogenic immune deficiency with alteration of T-cells function and favors EBV primary infection or reactivation of latent infection. This reduces the control of EBV-induced B-cell proliferation and probably leads to PTLD. Subsequent transformation into monoclonal proliferation is possible and may be due to chromosomic alterations (Hanto et al., 1983). This phenomenon is also observed in congenital or acquired (AIDS) immune deficiencies in which patients often develop lymphomas.

CLINICAL FEATURES

Two different types of clinical presentation are observed (Hanto et al., 1983). About 50% of the patients present with an infectious mononucleosis-like syndrome including fever, pharyngitis and widespraed lymphadenopathy. This form is more frequent in young patients, occurs early after transplant (few months) and is usually polyclonal. In the absence of adequate treatment, the disease may be rapidly lethal (Hanto et al., 1983 ; Renard et al., 1991). The other half of the patients develop a tumoral form of PTLD with localized solid tumor masses. This feature occurs preferentially in older patients, later after transplant (few years) and proliferation is often monoclonal (Hanto et al., 1983). Nodal involvement is more frequent in children, especially in the tonsils and adenoids (Stieber et al., 1991 ; Emond et al., 1990). PTLDs are also peculiar by a frequent extranodal involvement of 70% versus less than 50% in the general population (Penn, 1991). The organs involved include central nervous system, gastrointestinal tract (with possible perforation), lungs (Penn, 1991 ; Stieber et al., 1991 ; Emond et al., 1990) ; the graft itself may be the site of the proliferation in as many as 20% of the cases in liver recipients (Stieber et al., 1991).

PROGNOSIS AND TREATMENT

PTLDs have a severe prognosis and are associated with a 50-80% mortality within a few days or weeks (Stieber et al., 1991 ; Emond et al., 1990 ; Swinnen et al.,1990). Only 30% of deaths are directly due to PTLD, the most frequent cause of death being sepsis (Stieber et al., 1991 ; Emond et al., 1990 ; Swinnen et al.,1990). The frequency of septic complication in patients with PTLD suggests a high degree of immune deficiency in those patients.

However, recent data suggest that early diagnosis and appropriate therapy may improve the prognosis of PTLD.Therapeutic possibilities include reduction of immunosuppression, administration of acyclovir and surgery

Reduction of immunosuppression

Starzl et al. reported in 1984 the results of drastic reduction of cyclosporin by 60 to 100% (withdrawal of the drug). Cure of PTLD was obtained in 7 of 8 kidney recipients, 2 of 4 liver recipients and 2 of 5 heart recipients. This was not necessarily associated with irreversible rejection of the graft since 4 kidney, 2 liver and 2 heart recipients kept a functionnal graft.

Acyclovir

Acyclovir is a synthetic antiviral agent that blocks EBV DNA replication by inhibiting EBV-associated DNA polymerase. Its beneficial effect was shown by Hanto et al. in 1983, in patients with polyclonal PTLD associated with EBV infection. Two of 3 kidney recipients treated by reduction of immunosuppression and acyclovir were cured of PTLD but lost their graft ; another patients treated with acyclovir alone was cured and kept his graft. This emphasizes the importance of search for stigmata of EBV infection in patients with PTLDs, as well as the knowledge of EBV status prior to transplantation since acyclovir therapy might be indicated. However, monoclonal PTLDs were acyclovir resistant in Hanto's series (1983).

Role of Surgery

Stieber et al. (1991) from Pittsburgh emphasized recently the usefulness of surgery in the management of patients with PTLDs. This consisted in various diagnostic and therapeutic procedures including tonsillectomy, intestinal resection, solid organ resection, lymph node biopsy, exploratory laparotomy. Eleven of 23 patients treated by reduction of immunosuppression and acyclovir or interferon survived while all 11 patients treated by tumor resection alone (1 case) or associated with reduction of imunosuppression (5 cases) and acyclovir (5 cases) survived.

Place of chemotherapy

Indications of conventional antineoplastic chemotherapy in PTLD patients remain to be precised. It has been reported to be associated with worsening of the patients' condition and death (Starzl et al., 1984) and is advised against by the Pittsburgh group since it may increase immunodepression (Stieber et al., 1991)

CONCLUSIONS

The increasing incidence of PTLDs is probably the result of more powerful immnosuppressive regimens with a possible special effect of OKT3. The etiologic role of EBV is well established

The prognosis of PTLD is severe but it can be improved by : early diagnosis by surgical biopsy of the lesion, search for clonality and evidence of EBV infection and appropriate treatment including reduction of immunosuppression, acyclovir in case of EBV infection and surgical resection of tumor masses.

REFERENCES

Arnold, A., Cossman, J. et al. (1983) : Immunoglobulin-gene rearrangements as unique clonal markers in human lymphoid neoplasms. N. Engl. J. Med. 309, 1593-1599.

Emond, J.C., Heffron, T.G. et al. (1990) : Lymphoproliferative disorders after liver transplantation. A recent experience. H.P.B. Surgery 2 (suppl), 459.

Hanto, D.W., Gajl-Peczalska, K.J. et al. (1983) : Epstein-Barr virus (EBV) induced polyclonal and monoclonal B-cell lymphoproliferative diseases occurring afterrenal transplantation. Ann. Surg. 198, 356-368.

Ho, M., Jaffe, R. et al. (1988) : The frequency of Epstein-Barr virus infection and associated lymphoproliferative syndrome after transplantation and its manifestations in children. Transplantation. 45, 719-727

McKhann, C.F. (1969) : Primary malignancy in patients undergoing immunosuppression for renal transplantation Transplantation 8, 209-212.

Penn, I., Hammond, W. et al. (1969) : Malignant lymphomas in transplantation patients. Transplant. Proc. 1, 106-112.

Penn, I. (1991) : The changing pattern of posttransplant malignancies. Transplant. Proc. 23, 1101-1103.

Renard, T.H., Andrews, W.S. et al. (1991) : Relationship between OKT3, EBV seroconversion, and the lyphoproliferative syndrome in pediatric liver transplant recipients. Transplant. Proc. 23, 1473-1476.

Reyes, F. (1991) : Lymphome de Burkitt et lymphomes associés au virus d'Epstein-Barr. Modèles de lymphomogénèse. in Lymphomes non Hodgkiniens, eds. P. Solal-Céligny, N. Brousse, F. Reyes, C. Gisselbrecht, B. Coiffier, Paris, Frison-Roche.

Starzl, T.E., Nelesnik, M.A. et al. (1984) : Reversibility of lymphomas and lymphoproliferative lesions developing under cyclosporin-steroid therapy. Lancet i, 583-587.

Starzl, T.E., Rowe M.I. et al. (1989) : Transplantation of multiple abdominal viscera. J.A.M.A. 261, 1449-1457.

Stieber, A.C., Boillot, O. et al. (1991) : The surgical implications of the posttransplant lymphoproliferative disorders. Transplant. Proc. 23, 1477-1479

Swinnen, L.J., Costanzo-Nordin M.R. et al. (1990) : Increased incidence of lymphoproliferative disorder after immunosuppression with the monoclonal antibody OKT3 in cardiac-transplant recipients. N. Engl. J. Med. 323, 1723-1728.

Williams, J.W., Sankary, H.N. et al. (1989) : Splanchnic transplantation. An approach to the infant dependent on parenteral nutrition who develops irreversible liver disease. J.A.M.A. 261, 1458-1462.

> *Immunological, metabolic and infectious aspects of liver transplantation.* Eds D.A. Vuitton, C. Balabaud, D. Houssin, D. Dhumeaux. John Libbey Eurotext, Paris © 1991, pp. 91-96.

Recurrence of non-viral infectious diseases after liver transplantation

S. Bresson-Hadni[(1)]*, D. Lenys[(2)], J.P. Miguet[(1)], D.A. Vuitton[(1)], M.C. Becker[(1)], G. Landecy[(1)], G. Mantion[(1)], M. Gillet[(1)]

[(1)] *Groupe de Recherche en Transplantation Hépatique et Immunologie Clinique, boulevard Fleming, CHU Jean Minjoz, 25030 Besançon Cedex, France.* [(2)] *Laboratoire de Cytologie-cytogénétique, Faculté de Médecine, 25030 Besançon, France*

* *Author for correspondence*

SUMMARY

Currently, the unique non viral infectious liver disease which has constituted an indication of liver transplantation (OLT) is incurable alveolar echinococcosis (AE) of the liver due to the proliferation of the larvae of *Echinococcus multilocularis*. Twenty one OLT have been performed in Europe for this rare parasitic disease. True recurrence on the graft has been reported in only one case. On the 17 AE patients transplanted in our center, 14 have survived after the 3rd month. In order to detect any recurrences at an early stage, serial morphological and immunological investigations were performed after OLT. Specific IgG levels as well as specific cellular immunity were evaluated using ELISA and a lymphocyte proliferation test respectively. None of these patients had a true recurrence of AE within a mean follow-up period of 30 months (rage 9-48). However, in 6 cases, OLT had to be considered as a palliative procedure due to the presence of persistent parasitic foci (pulmonar and/or hepatic). In these 6 patients, who remained asymptomatic during the whole follow-up, the growth of the residual parasitic foci was apparent and the specific humoral and even cellular immunological parameters increased significantly despite the immunosuppressive therapy. Immunological parameters decreased significantly and became negative in all the other patients but 2 who are currently followed-up very carefully.

To our knowledge, the only non-viral infectious disease which has constitute an indication of orthotopic liver transplantation (OLT) is incurable alveolar echinococcosis (AE) of the liver. This uncommon parasitic disease caused by the chronic proliferation of the larvae of a small cestode, *Echinococcus multilocularis,* is endemic in Central Europe (Southern Germany, Western Austria, Switzerland and Eastern France), in most of the Soviet Union, in Japan and in North America (MIGUET & BRESSON-HADNI, 1989). The very slow progression of the disease and its possible invasion of the biliary tract and/or hepatic vessels and/or the inferior vena cava are the main characteristics of this severe disease which is often compared to a liver cancer. Currently, due to the lack of parasitolytic drugs, surgery remains the only efficient treatment of AE. However, at the time of diagnosis, a curative partial hepatectomy is feasible in only 40 % of the cases. In the remaining 60 %, only palliative procedures or OLT are possible (CHAPUIS et al. 1987, MIGUET & BRESSON-HADNI, 1989, BRESSON-HADNI et al. 1991). Since 1986, about 20 OLT for AE have been performed in France, 17 of them in Besançon (BRESSON-HADNI et al. 1991).The aim of this paper is to provide some preliminary information about the possibility of recurrence of AE after OLT.

First, a distinction has to be made between true recurrence after radical OLT and the evolution of parasitic foci left after palliative OLT and/or parasitic metastases. During the last

5 years, 21 OLT were performed in France for AE. A true recurrence in the liver graft was observed in only one case, whereas the persistence of residual parasitic tissue was discovered in 7 cases (Table 1). Out of 3 patients transplanted for this indication in Nancy, one had neurological symptoms 6 months post-OLT associated with an increase of specific antibodies (P. BOISSEL, personal communication). A cerebral CT-scan was performed and showed a parasitic metastasis. It was not possible to determine when the brain metastasis occurred because a pre-OLT cerebral CT-scan had not been done. After administration of an oral therapy with the parasitostatic benzimidazole drug, mebendazole, the clinical symptoms disappeared and the parasitic lesion remained unchanged during the next 6 months of follow-up. In Clermont-Ferrand (J. CHIPPONI, personal communication), a true recurrence in the grafted liver occurred in one of two transplanted AE patients in this center. This patient received an OLT for a severe AE of the liver, associated with peritoneal and splenic metastases. Two months post-OLT, he experienced a septic shock which was promptly related to a recurrent parasitic liver abscess in the right lobe. In fact, the histological examination of this lesion revealed multiple small typical parasitic vesicles which evoked an hematogenic dissemination. This may be due to the splenic metastasis which could not be removed during OLT for technical reasons. A percutaneous drainage associated with antibiotics and parasitostatic chemotherapy with albendazole was effective : the parasitic lesion has remained unchanged with a current follow-up of 18 months.

Table 1 : RECURRENCE OF ALVEOLAR ECHINOCOCCOSIS (AE) AFTER LIVER TRANSPLANTATION

Center	n of OLT for AE*	Follow-up	recurrence	Localization
Paris-Cochin (France)	1	48 mo	0	-
Nancy (France)	3	12 mo	1	cerebral+
Strasbourg (France)	1	30 mo	0	-
Besançon (France)	14	30 mo	6	pulmonar and/or peri hepatic **
Clermont (France)	2	18 mo	1	liver graft

* survival > 3 mo.   + no pre-OLT cerebral CT-scan
** present at the time of OLT

In Besançon, 14 out of the 17 transplanted AE patients have survived after the third post-operative month (BRESSON-HADNI et al. 1991). They underwent serial morphological and specific immunological investigations to detect a parasitic recurrence at an early stage. None of these 14 patients had a true recurrence of AE on the liver graft within a mean follow-up period of 30 months (range 9-48). However, in 6 of the 14 patients, OLT had to be considered as a palliative procedure : in fact, these patients had persistent pulmonar metastases and/or residual peri-hepatic parasitic foci (noticed by the surgeon) after OLT. In the 8 remaining patients, OLT was considered as "curative".

To assess specific humoral immunity, an ELISA test detecting specific IgG was performed. Three parasitic antigens were used : a crude *E. multilocularis* (*Emc* Ag), a crude *E. granulosus* (*Eg*) Ag and the highly specific antigenic fraction *Em2* (GOTTSTEIN et al. 1989). This serology was done before OLT, 1 month post-OLT and then every 3 months. Specific cellular immunity, which plays a major role in this disease (BRESSON-HADNI et al. 1989 a), was evaluated with a lymphocyte proliferation test using a crude *Emc* Ag according to a technique previously described (BRESSON-HADNI et al. 1989 a). This test was carried out before OLT, 3 months post-OLT and then every 6 months.

In spite of the triple immuno-suppressive therapy (steroïds, cyclosporine and azathioprine), the specific humoral and even cellular immunological parameters, enabled us to distinguish between "palliative" and "curative" OLT. In fact, in the six patients with an incomplete eviction of the parasitic disease, a marked increase of anti-*Emc* and anti-*Eg* IgG was observed after a transient decrease during the first 3 post-operative months (Fig. 1A). However, IgG directed against *Em2* Ag remained undetectable until the end of the 2nd or the 3rd year of follow-up (Fig.1A). A similar evolution was observed in 2 of the 8 patients with a surgically documented curative OLT (Fig. 1B). In the 6 remaining patients, specific IgG disappeared within the first months post-OLT and remained undetectable during the whole follow-up (Fig. 1C).

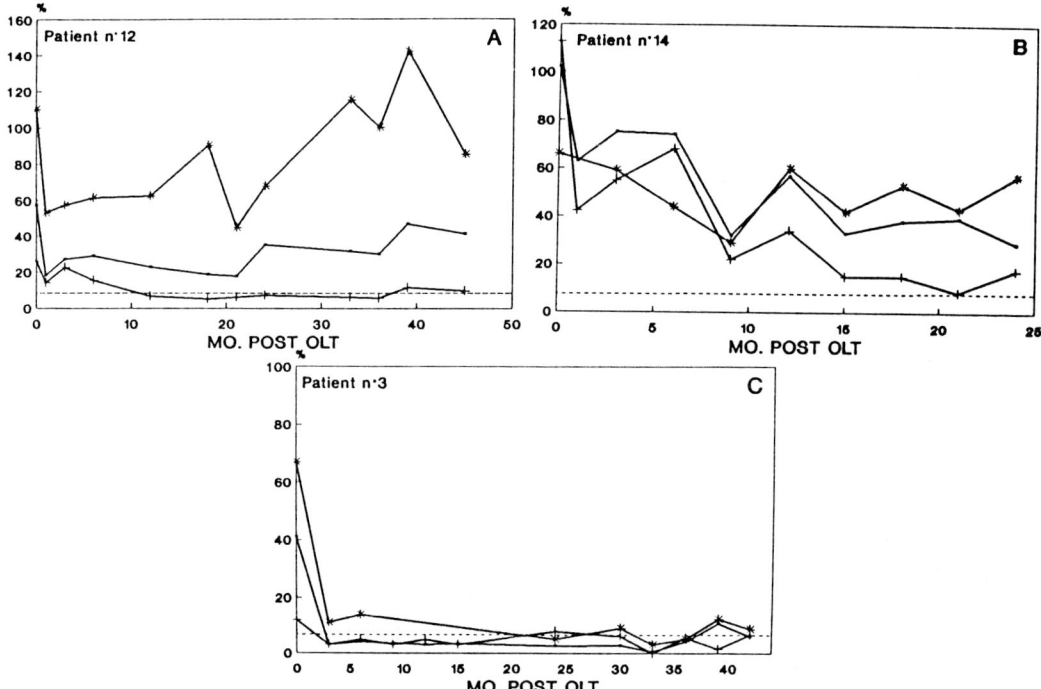

Fig. I. Evolution of specific IgG after OLT in 3 transplanted AE patients. Patient with a "palliative" OLT (A) : Initial decrease followed by a subsequent increase of IgG against Eg Ag (***) since the end of the first year of follow-up. IgG against Emc Ag (-•-•-) also increased but later and lower. Persistent negativation of the IgG against Em2 Ag (-+-+-). (B) : Patient with an apparently "curative" OLT : the evolution was similar to that of the "palliative" group but so far the morphological investigations have not confirmed the recurrence of AE. (C) : Evolutive pattern of specific IgG in a patient having undergone a "radical" OLT : rapid and persistent negativation of the antibodies directed against the 3 parasitic antigens.

In all 14 patients, the specific lymphocyte sensitization decreased during the first 6 months post-OLT, probably due to the high dosages of the immunosuppressive drugs given at that time. However, this specific lymphocyte sensitization reappeared later, even in the "radical" group (Fig. 2 A-C). In this group, the disappearance of specific lymphocyte sensitization finally occurred in 6 out of 8 cases between 24 to 48 months after OLT (Fig. 2C). Interestingly, in the two patients with increased specific humoral immunity, a parallel increase of the specific cellular immunity was observed after the first year of follow-up (Fig. 2B). However, so far, these 2 patients are completely asymptomatic, and all morphological investigations (successive abdominal, thoracic and, in one case, cerebral CT-scan) remain normal.

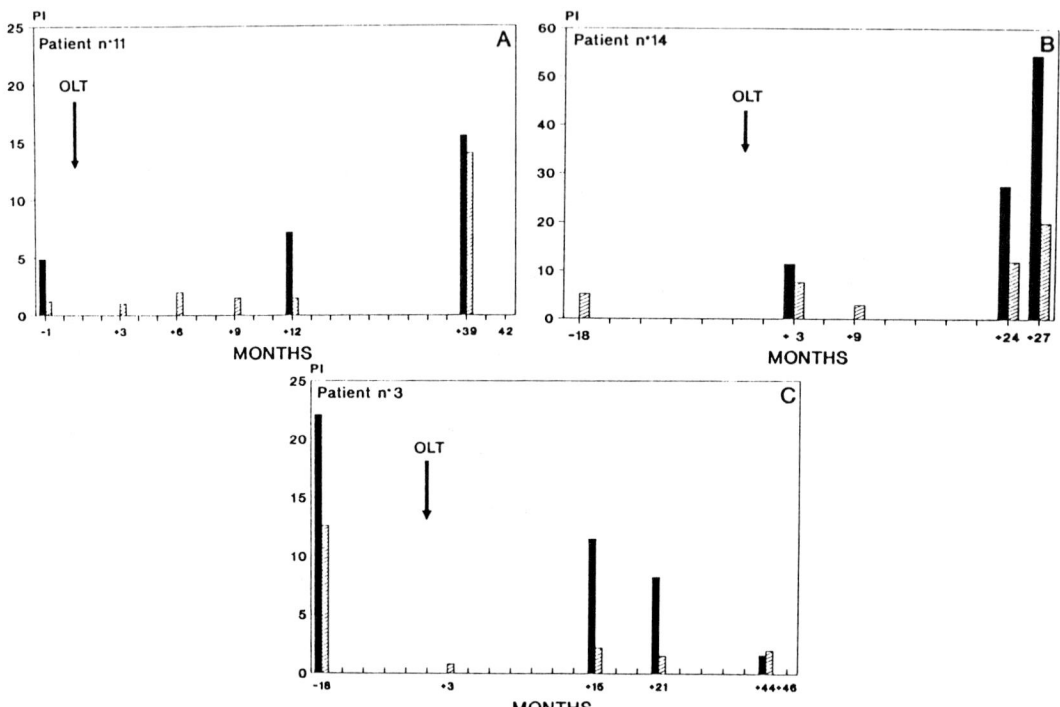

Fig. II. Evolution of specific lymphocyte sensitization after OLT in 3 transplanted AE patients. The proliferative index (PI) was significant for any value > 3 with Emc Ag 50 μg/ml (■) and > 2 with Emc Ag 5 μg/ml (▨). (A) : Patient having had a "palliative" OLT. Transient PI decrease during the first post-operative months and intensification 3 years after OLT. (B) : Patient with an apparently "curative" OLT but showing the same evolution of specific lymphocyte sensitization as in the palliative group. (C) : Evolution in a patient having had a "curative" OLT : the disappearance of the specific lymphocyte sensitization finally occurred during the 3rd year of follow-up.

In the six patients with a confirmed "palliative" OLT and who remained asymptomatic during the whole follow-up, the growth of the residual parasitic foci was apparent on successive morphological investigations, but was relatively slow (Fig. 3 A-B). However, this increase in size, over such a short period of time and particularly in the lungs, is uncommon. In our experience, AE pulmonar metastases in non liver transplanted AE patients are remarkably stable during a long follow-up period, sometimes exceeding ten years (BRESSON-HADNI et al. 1989 b). Consequently, the role of immunosuppressive therapy on the growth of metastases has to be raised. Preliminary results on a murine model of peritoneal AE support this hypothesis (M. LIANCE, personal communication).

Four out of the six patients with "palliative" OLT were given albendazole therapy during the second year of follow-up, when the graft function was stable. We prefer not to treat them earlier because of the lack of information about possible pharmacological interactions between these compounds and the immunosuppressive drugs. In 2 patients, this treatment had to be promptly withdrawn because of a rapid increase of transaminases.

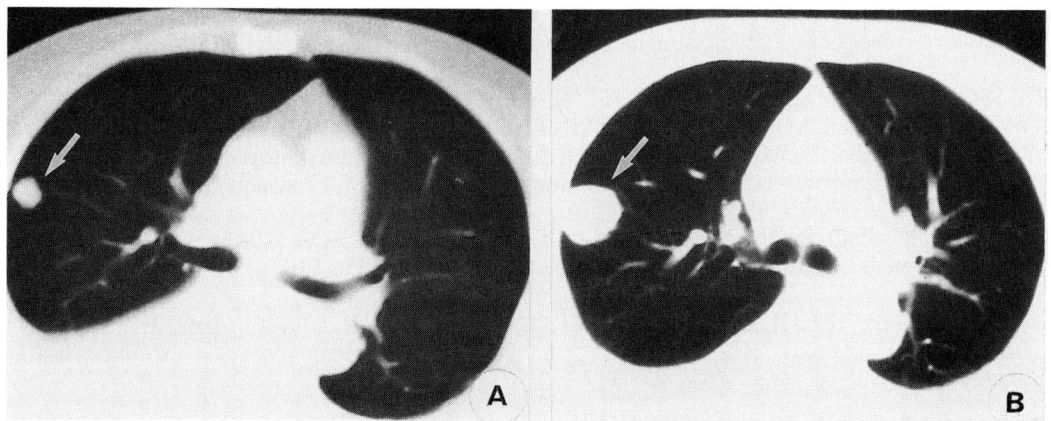

Fig. III. CT-scan evolution of a parasitic pulmonar metastasis (arrow) under immunosuppression : before OLT (A) and 42 months post-OLT (B).

In conclusion, true recurrence is possible in transplanted AE patients but is probably exceptional, according to our experience. Persistant parasitic foci residues may increase in size after OLT but are well tolerated by the patients, at least in such a middle term follow-up. The combined study of the evolution of specific humoral and cellular immunity appears useful to distinguish between "palliative" and "radical" OLT. Moreover, it could be useful in predicting a recurrence of the parasitic disease. The immunological tests of poor specificity, but high sensitivity, (using crude heterologous and/or homologous antigens) seem to be better diagnostic tools than the most sophisticated test using a high specific antigenic fraction (*Em2*). Progress has to be made a) to specify the role of immunosuppression on *E. multilocularis* growth and b) to better define possible interactions between benzimidazoles and immunosuppressive drugs.

ACKNOWLEDGEMENTS :

We wish to thank Prof. J. CHIPPONI, Prof. P. BOISSEL, Prof. D. HOUSSIN and Prof. P. WOLF for kindly providing information about the liver transplanted AE patients in their centers and Mrs Pamela ALBERT and Annie GROSPERRIN for the preparation of the manuscript.

REFERENCES

BRESSON-HADNI, S., VUITTON, D.A., LENYS, D., LIANCE, M., MIGUET, J.P. (1989 a) : Cellular immune response in *Echinococcus multilocularis* infection in humans : 1) lymphocyte reactivity to *Echinococcus*
antigens in patients with alveolar echinococcosis. *Clin. Exp. Immunol.* 78, 61-66.

BRESSON-HADNI, S., VUITTON, D.A., DIDIER, D., ETIEVENT, J.P., MANTION, G., MIGUET, J.P., GILLET, M. (1989 b) : Métastases pulmonaires de l'échinococcose alvéolaire : fréquence et mécanismes de survenue. *Presse Méd.* (lettre) 18, 83.

BRESSON-HADNI, S., FRANZA, A., MIGUET, J.P., VUITTON, D.A., LENYS, D, MONNET, E., LANDECY, G., PAINTAUD, G., ROHMER, P., BECKER, M.C., CHRISTOPHE, J.L., MANTION, G., GILLET, M. (1991) : Orthotopic liver transplantation for incurable alveolar echinococcosis of the liver : report of 17 cases. *Hepatology.* in press.

CHAPUIS, Y., HOUSSIN, D., BROUZES, S., ORTEGA, D. (1987) : Transplantation hépatique dans l'échinococcose alvéolaire. *Chirurgie* 113. 634-640.

GOTTSTEIN, B., TSCHUDI, K., ECKERT, J., AMMANN, R. (1989) : Em2-ELISA for the follow-up of alveolar echinococcosis after complete surgical resection of liver lesions. *Transact. Roy. Trop. Med. Hyg.* 83, 389-393.

MIGUET, J.P. & BRESSON-HADNI, S. (1989) : Alveolar echinococcosis of the liver. *J. Hepatol.* 8, 373-379.

Does primary biliary cirrhosis recur after liver transplantation ?

James Neuberger, Stefan Hubscher *

*The Liver Unit, The Queen Elizabeth Hospital, Edgbaston, Birmingham, B15 2TH, UK. * Department of Pathology, University of Birmingham, Medical school, Birmingham, UK*

Primary Biliary Cirrhosis (PBC) is one of the commonest indications for liver transplantation in Europe. In 1982, we reported three patients in whom we suggested the disease had recurred in the allograft (Neuberger et al 1982). The interpretation of the findings has been questioned and the possible recurrence of the disease in the allograft has since been the subject of considerable controversy (Jones 1982, Van Thiel and Gavaler 1987).

Diagnosis of Primary Biliary Cirrhosis

In the ungrafted patient, the diagnosis of primary biliary cirrhosis is based on a combination of clinical, serological and histological features. Routine liver tests show the presence of biliary disease but the demonstration of a raised serum immunoglobulins (especially IgM) and the presence of antimitochondrial antibodies allow the diagnosis to be made more readily. Indeed, the presence of M2 subtype of antimitochondrial antibodies or the presence of antibodies to the pyruvate dehydrogenase complex may be pathognomonic of the disease (Gershwin et al 1988, Mitchison et al 1986). Furthermore, both in vivo and in vitro studies show widespread disturbance of the immune cellular and humoral systems. For a formal diagnosis, histology is usually required and this will show features of non-suppurative destructive cholangitis. Even histology will not always show pathognomonic features of this disease. PBC is associated with the development of auto-immune diseases such as the Sicca Syndrome, Raynaud's Phenomenon, the CREST syndrome and thyroid disorders.

The pathogenesis of the disease remains uncertain. It is not yet established whether the antimitochondrial antibodies, highly specific for the disease, are associated with the pathogenesis or merely reflect a host abnormality. On the one hand, immunisation of a wide variety of laboratory animals with purified E2 (the main epitope of pyruvate dehydrogenase complex, the antigen recognised by AMA) whilst leading to the appearance of anti-mitochondrial antibodies in the serum, is not associated with any evidence of liver damage (Krams et al 1989a). On the other hand, immunisation of severe combined immunodeficient mice (SCID mice) with lymphocytes from patients with PBC is associated with a far greater incidence of bile duct damage reminiscent of PBC than when the mice were immunised with lymphocytes from normal humans (Krams et al 1989b).

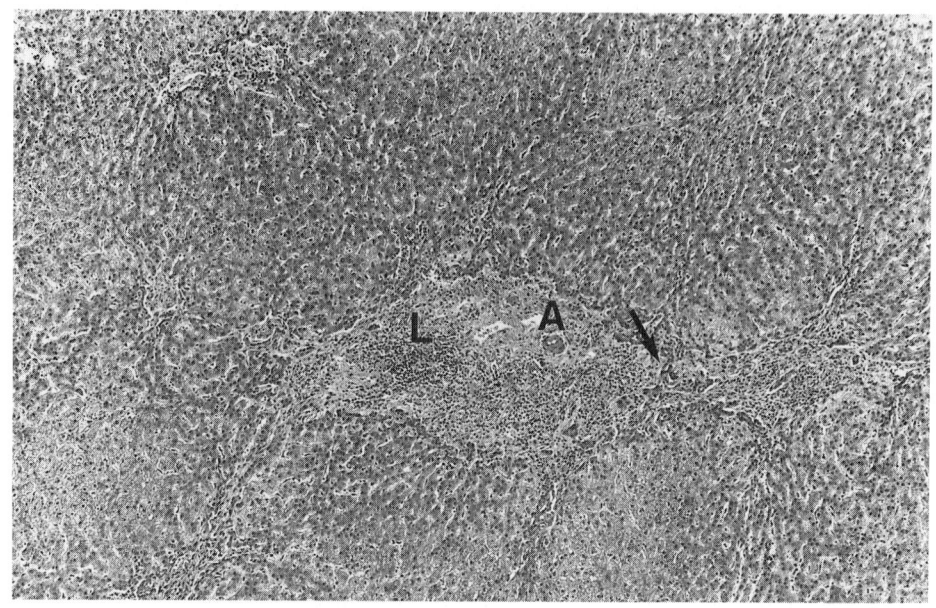

Fig (1)   Hepatectomy PBC. There is a vanishing bile duct syndrome with an unaccompanyied artery (A). Portal tracts show fibrous expansion and marginal ductular proliferation (arrowed). L = lymphoid aggregate.

Abnormalities of immune function, which persist after transplantation, may represent underlying host abnormalities which indicates a predisposition to the disease; normalisation of abnormalities may be a consequence of the immunosuppression improving lymphocyte abnormalities (Al-Aghbar et al 1986). Possibly the gold standard for the diagnosis, namely histology, is complicated by the finding that many patients post-transplant have abnormal allograft histology (Hubscher 1990) and rejection is characterised by an immune attack on the bile ducts. Thus, the diagnosis of recurrent PBC after transplantation has to be made by considering the whole patient, clinical, serological and histological.

Clinical Features of PBC Recurrence

After the initial report suggesting recurrence of PBC (Neuberger et al 1982), the Cambridge/King's College Hospital series was followed up and a subsequent analysis appeared in 1989 (Polson et al 1989). In this analysis 23 patients who had survived more than a year after transplantation were analysed. Of these 23 patients, 9 survived for more than 2 year and 6 for five years. Nineteen were alive at the time of the analysis. One year after transplantation, all patients were free of pruritus and lethargy. Raynaud's phenomenon had improved and Sicca syndrome was symptomatically improved in 9 of 11 patients. 4 lost all symptoms (Table 1).

Table 1
Clinical Features of PBC
Before and After Transplantation in 23 Patients
(Polson et al 1990)

Symptoms	Number	Resolved	Recurred	De Novo Development
Pruritus	20	15	5	-
Sicca	11	4 (5 improved)	-	2
Raynaud's	12	4 (7 improved)	-	1
Hypothyroidism	-	-	-	-

Pruritus recurred in 5. De novo development of Raynaud's phenomenon occurred in one patient, Sicca syndrome in 2 patients and sclerodactyly in 2 patients. 2 patients developed biochemical evidence of hypothyroidism. Thus, it would appear that the transplant and consequent immunosuppression does not completely abolish the propensity of patients who suffer from PBC to develop some of the associated extra-hepatic syndromes. Modification of diseased processes by immunosuppression, in particular Cyclosporin, cannot be excluded. This, of course, does not show conclusively that PBC recurs after transplantation

Serological Features of PBC

The classical abnormalities of standard liver tests in PBC are that of cholestasis. There are many causes of cholestasis in patients post transplant, including cholangitis, biliary tract outflow obstruction and rejection. Thus, it is very difficult to make any useful deduction from the standard liver tests.

More specific are the levels of serum IgM and the antimitochondrial antibodies. In the King's College Hospital/ Addenbrooke's series (Polson et al 1989), there was a significant fall in serum IgM levels. In all patients but 1, IgM was elevated prior to transplantation and fell to within the normal range in 2 others. Anti-mitochondrial antibodies, were initially detectable in all patients prior to grafting with a median titre of 1 in 640. At the most recent time of testing after transplantation 1 to 10 years later, AMA were detectable in all 19 albeit at a slightly lower titre. However, in four patients studied sequentially with time there was a progressive increase in the anti-mitochondrial antibodies. Our own data (Neuberger, unpublished) suggest that AMA are of the anti-M2 titre and this was confirmed by others (Haagsma et al 1987). The Dutch group found, as we had, that a small number of patients lose antibody entirely although it is possible that with prolonged follow up, titres may once more start to rise.

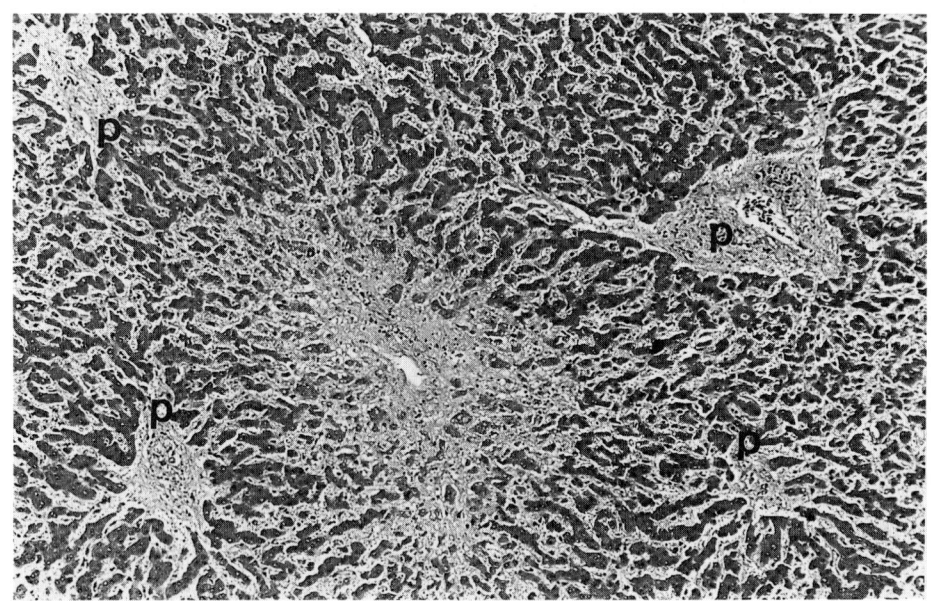

Fig (2). End-stage Chronic Rejection - autopsy specimen. 4 portal tracts (p) and without bile ducts. There is no significant inflammation or fibrosis and no ductular proliferatiron. The liver/parenchyma shows perivenular hepatocyte dropout and fibrosis.

Analysis of the in vitro immunological abnormalities in PBC is almost impossible to interpret since all patients are, of necessity, on immunosuppression and this in vivo will clearly affect lymphocyte abnormality tested in vitro.

Histological Features

The main histological features of PBC and allograft rejection have been documented by a number of authoritative sources and are summarised in Table 2 and compared with chronic rejection.

Table 2
Features of PBC and Allograft Rejection

Histological Feature	Chronic Rejection Early	Late	P.B.C Early	Late
(A) PORTAL TRACTS				
(1) Bile Ducts				
Bile Duct Damage[1]	+++	- →+	++/+++	+ ++
Bile Duct Loss	+/-	+++	+	++
(2) Inflammation				
Chronic inflammatory infiltrate	+++	- →+	++	++
Lymphoid follicles	-	-	+	+
Granulomas	-	-	++	+
(3) Vascular Lesions				
Arterial foam cells/ fibrosis	- →+[2]	+++	-	-
Venous endothelial inflammation	+ +++	+/-	-	-
(4) Secondary Changes				
Bile ductular proliferation	-	-	+	+++
Fibrosis	-	+/-	+	++ +++
(B) PARENCHYMA				
(5) Cholestasis				
Severity	++/+++	+++	- +	+++
Distribution	p.v.	p.v.	p.p.	pp+pv
(6) Hepatocyte Necrosis/Fibrosis				
Perivenular	+	++	-	-
(7) C.A.P	0	0	+	+++

1 active lesions 2 rarely affects small vessels sampled in needle biopsies. PP periportal, PV perivenous, CAP - copper associated protein

Although there are some similarities and shared findings, such as bile duct damage, there are certain features such as bile duct proliferation and granulomas, which are found in PBC and not in rejection. (Fig 1 and 2).

Both conditions share features of bile duct damage and loss with central cholestasis. Chronic rejection is characterised by arterial lesions (Fig.2) often with foamy macrophages extending into the liver parenchyma. Granulomas, a feature particularly of early and benign PBC are occasionally seen in late PBC but not in chronic rejection. In the Polson series (1989) liver biopsies taken one year after transplantation showed some histological features of PBC (Table 3).

Table 3
Histological Features of Bile Duct Damage
(Polson et al 1989)

Copper Associated Protein*	4
Granulomas	3
Ductular Proliferation	6
Lymphoid Aggregates	8

* In absence of cholestasis

In comparison, 102 patients grafted for conditions other than PBC who had survived for more than a year were studied and of these 50 had had liver biopsies. 12 of these 50 patients had bile duct changes apparent on the biopsies taken more than one year later. The clinical or histological diagnoses varied from cytomegalovirus infection to venous outflow block, ascending cholangitis, chronic rejection, chronic active or chronic persistent hepatitis. Thus, in all cases alternative clinical and histological diagnoses were apparent from the history or investigations. None of the patients had any symptoms or biochemical abnormalities suggestive or compatible with a diagnosis of recurrent PBC.

In our own series in Birmingham annual liver biopsies are performed on all liver transplant recipients and preliminary results of this analysis has shown a high incidence of abnormalities in the graft despite normal liver function tests (Hubscher 1990). Preliminary analysis of 15 patients with PBC (Buist et al 1989) showed that there were many lesions consistent with PBC recurrence in that group. Again the histological probability of recurrence of disease was shown only in a small proportion of patients transplanted for PBC (Fig 3 and 4).

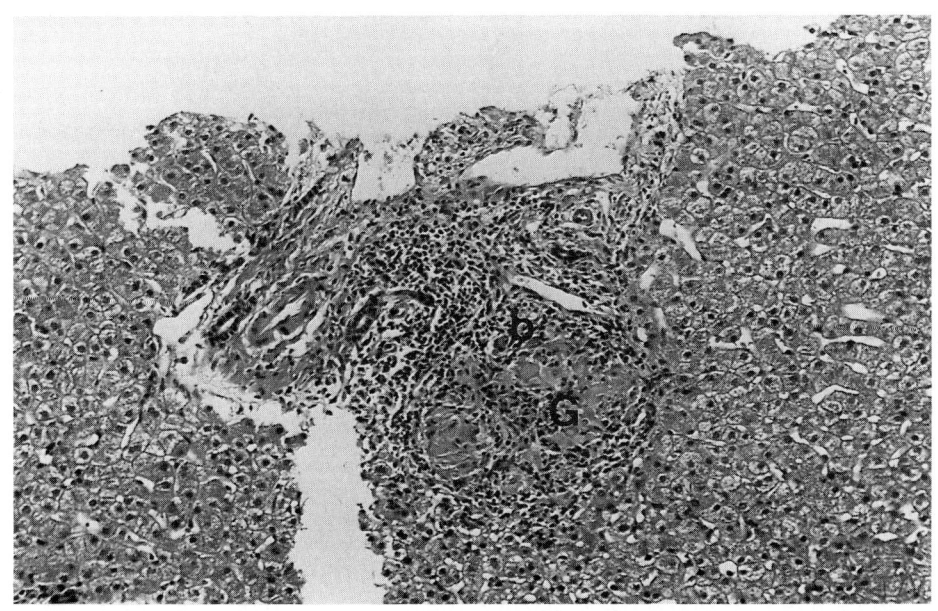

Fig (3). Early recurrent PBC in liver allograft. Biopsy taken 12 months post-transplant showing a portal tract granuloma (G) adjacent to a small bile duct (B).

The literature contains only one other report known to these authors that PBC may recur in the graft (Dietz et al 1990). This Austrian group reported analysis of 8 patients grafted for PBC with a mean survival of 27 months.

In 2 patients, there were features of recurrent PBC with evidence of granulomas and bile duct damage.

Evidence Against Recurrence

There have been two major papers from Starzl's group (Demetris et al 1988 and Esquivel et al 1988) and one from Fennell et al 1983 which have been quoted as showing lack of recurrence of PBC after transplantation. The paper by Demetris consisted of a retrospective histopathological review of all pathological specimens taken from failed transplant recipients. They also compared the histological features of end-stage PBC with failed allografts. Of the 394 patients grafted from 1981 to July 1986, 106 were for PBC. Mitochondrial antibodies were present in 98% prior to transplantation and in 42 of the 45 one year survivors.

The authors confirm that there were significant differences between chronic rejection and end-stage primary biliary cirrhosis. The authors also state that there were no features allowing them to diagnose recurrence of PBC in the allograft. In the companion paper by Esquivel, clinical features as well as histological features were analysed.

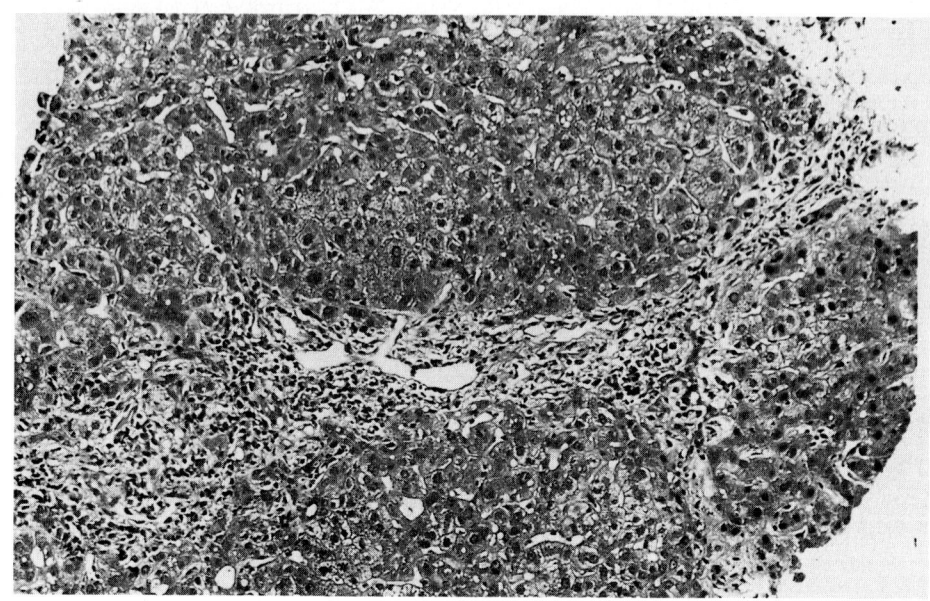

Fig (4). Recurrent PBC in Liver Allograft - Progressive Damage. Biopsy taken 36 months post-transplant (same case of Fig 3) shows secondary damages in portal tracts with fibrous expansion, marginal ductular proliferation and early portal-portal linkage.

Biopsies were analysed from 2 months post-operatively but only failed allografts were assessed. Of the 52 surviving patients, 13 had some abnormality of liver function but in all cases this was of a minor degree. Although none of the features on histology showed evidence of recurrent PBC, of the 8 patients who had liver biopsies, in most cases these were taken within the first few months of transplantation. In only two cases this was in more than one year and in one of these features on histology were of acute rejection. Again, Haagsma et al (1987) was unable to find evidence of recurrence amongst 9 patients in biopsies which were done yearly for up to five years.

What Conclusions Can Be Drawn?

How then can these two opposing views be combined? There seems to be little doubt that the serological and extra-hepatic features of PBC may persist, recur or develop de novo after transplantation but this does not prove recurrence of PBC in the allograft. The King's/Cambridge data suggests that histological features of PBC are present in only a proportion of allograft recipients. This might explain why in the comparatively small number of patients reported from Germany and the Netherlands studied, no features of recurrent disease were observed. In contrast, the Pittsburgh experience is more difficult to reconcile. Nevertheless, one possible difference is that is appears that biopsies were taken only for specific indications such as failed allografts. Thus, any features of non-suppurative destructive cholangitis may be masked by chronic rejection, infection or ischaemia. Patients in King's/Cambridge and in Birmingham who underwent biopsies as part of a protocol assessment rather than when abnormalities of liver function suggested significant disease.

In almost every case the liver showed features only of early disease. Perhaps it is not surprising that for a disease which presents in the middle years of life, that features of recurrence are not apparent within the first few years after transplantation.

Implication for Patients

With the exception of one patient who died with cirrhosis at 9 years post grafting, documentation of recurrent disease in the allograft remains of academic interest only and appears to have little effect on the clinical wellbeing of the patient. The drugs commonly used for immunosuppression, Azathioprine, Corticosteroids and Cyclosporin A all have an effect in slowing the progression of the disease. Thus, immunosuppression may modify the natural history of the disease.

If it is accepted that PBC does recur in the allograft, does this lead to any information about the pathogenesis of the enigmatic disease? The answer, regrettably, is no. A number of hypotheses have been suggested for the pathogenesis of the disease: these include an infective agent, abnormality of host T-cells, a modified graft versus host disease. Recurrence of viral disease in the allograft is well described for viral hepatitis types A, B C and D. Host abnormalities may be affected by immunosuppression but as the intrinsic host abnormalities are not yet defined, this cannot be explored in great detail. The only hypothesis that would be excluded by recurrence of disease in the graft is an intrinsic host dependant abnormality of the middle sized intra-hepatic ducts.

No doubt with greater follow up and more meticulous attention to histology and the greater use of protocol biopsies in patients who are otherwise well and asymptomatic, the natural history of the allograft in PBC recipients can be studied and a true likelihood of recurrence finally established.

REFERENCES

Al-Aghbar, M.N.A. Alexander,.G. Neuberger J. et al (1986): The effect of prednisolone in vitro on immunoglobulin production in Primary Biliary Cirrhosis. Clin. Exp. Immunol. 66, 663-670.

Buist L.J. Hubscher, S. Vickers, C. Michell I. Neuberger, J. McMaster, P. (1989): Does liver transplantation cure Primary Biliary Cirrhosis? Transplantation Proceedings. 21, 2402.

Demetris, A.J. Markus, B.H. Esquivel, C. et al (1988): Pathologic analysis of liver transplantation for primary biliary cirrhosis. Hepatology. 8, 937-947.

Dietze, O. Vogel, W. Malgreiter, R. (1990): Primary biliary cirrhosis after liver transplantation. Transplantation Proceedings. 22, 1501-1502.

Equivel, C. Van Thiel, D. Demetris, AJ. et al (1988): Transplantation for primary biliary cirrhosis. Gastroenterology. 94, 1207-1216.

Fennell, R.H. Shikes, R.H. Vierling, J.M. (1983): Relationship of pre-transplant hepatobiliary disease to bile duct damage occuring in the liver allograft. Hepatology. 3, 84-89.

Gershwin, M.E. Coppel, R.L. McKay, I.R. (1988): Primary biliary cirrhosis and mitochondrial autoantigen. Hepatology. 8, 147-151.

Haagsma, E.B. Manns, M. Klein, R. et al (1987): Subtypes of antimitochondrial antibodies in primary biliary cirrhosis before and after orthotopic liver transplantation. Hepatology. 7, 129- 133.

Hubscher, S. (1990): Chronic hepatitis in the liver allograft. Hepatology. 12, 1257-1254.

Jones, E.A. (1982): Primary biliary cirrhosis and liver transplantation. N.Engl.J.Med. 306, 41-43.

Krams, S.M. Dorskind, K. Gershwin, ME. (1989b): Generation of biliary lesions after transfer of human lymphocytes into severe combined immunodeficient (SCID) mice. J.Exp.Med. 170, 1919-1930.

Krams, S.M. Surh, C. Coppel, R. et al (1989a): Immunisation of experimental animals with dihydrolipoamide acetyltransferase as a purified recombinant polypeptide, generates mitochondrial antibodies but not primary biliary cirrhosis. Hepatology. 9, 411-416.

Mitchison, H.C. Bassendine, M.C. Hendrick A et al (1986): Positive antimitochondrial antibody but normal alkaline phosphatases. Is this primary biliary cirrhosis? Hepatology. 6, 1279-1284.

Neuberger, J. Portmann, B. MacDougall, B. Calne, R.Y. Williams, R. (1982): Recurrence of primary biliary cirrhosis after liver transplantation. New.Eng.Journ.Med. 306, 1-4.

Polson, R.J. Portmann, B. Neuberger, J. Calne, R.Y. Williams, R. (1989): Evidence for disease recurrence after liver transplantation for primary biliary cirrhosis. Gastroenterology. 97, 715-725.

Van Thiel, D.H. Gavaler, J. (1987): Recurrent disease in patient with liver transplantation: when does it occur and how can we be sure? Hepatology. 7, 181-183.

Author index

Adams D.H., 43

Bach J.F., 11
Balabaud C., 17
Becker M.C., 91
Bioulac-Sage P., 17
Böker K., 65
Bresson-Hadni S., 59, 91

Caillat-Zucman S., 11
Calmus Y., 35
Canioni P., 17
Carles J., 17
Cherqui D., 83

Dussaix E., 77

Farle M., 65

Gallis J.L., 17
Gillet M., 59, 91
Gubernatis G., 65

Höckerstedt K., 49
Houssin D., 35
Hubscher S., 97

Janvier G., 17

Kantelip B., 59
Klein H., 65
Kreis H., 11

Landecy G., 91
Lautenschlager I., 49
Lautz H.U., 65
Legendre C., 11
Lenys D., 91

Magnette J., 59
Mantion G., 59, 91
Miguet J.P., 59, 91
Müller R., 65

Neuberger J., 97
Niehoff G., 65
Noël L.H., 11

Pichlmayr R., 65

Seilles E., 59
Stangel W., 65
Steinhoff G., 27

Tongio M.M., 1
Tovey M., 11
Tusch G., 65

Vanden Broecke C., 11
Vanlemmens C., 59
Vuitton D.A., 59, 91

Wittekind C., 65

LOUIS-JEAN
avenue d'Embrun, 05003 GAP cedex
Tél. : 92.53.17.00
Dépôt légal : 721 — Septembre 1991
Imprimé en France